EALTH PROMOTION IN MIDWIFERY

HEALTH PROMOTION IN MIDWIFERY

Principles and Practice

By

Helen Crafter MSc RGN RM FP Cert ADM PGCEA,
Senior Lecturer in Midwifery,
Thames Valley University,
London, UK

with contributing chapters from:

Patricia Wilson
Val Thomas
Maggie McNab
Lea Jamieson and Louise M. Long
and
Margaret Adams

A member of the Hodder Headline Group
LONDON SYDNEY AUCKLAND

First published in Great Britain in 1997 by
Arnold, a member of the Hodder Headline Group
338 Euston Road, London, NW1 3BH

British Library Cataloguing in Publication Data
A catalogue record for this book is available from the British Library

Library of Congress Cataloging-in-Publication Data
A catalog record for this book is available from the Library of Congress

ISBN 0 340 61473 0

Composition in 10/12pt Palatino by Photoprint Typesetters, Torquay, Devon
Printed and bound in Great Britain by JW Arrowsmith Ltd, Bristol

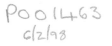

I would like to dedicate this book to my mother, Nancy Crafter, who showered me with encouragement as I started writing but sadly has not lived to see its completion, and my daughter, Oriana Nancy Hine, who made her appearance halfway through and continued the encouragement in her own special way.

Contents

List of contributors

Margaret Adams MBE, MSc, RGN, RM, MTD, DN
Associate Lecturer, European Institute of Health and Medical Sciences, University of Surrey, formerly Head of Midwifery Education, Thames Valley University, UK

Helen Crafter MSc, RGN, RM, FP Cert, ADM, PGCEA
Senior Lecturer in Midwifery, Thames Valley University, London, UK

Lea Jamieson MSc, BEd (Hons), RGN, RM, MTD
Independent Midwifery Education Consultant and Midwifery Education Advisor for KCL, formerly Head of Midwifery and Women's Health Studies, Nightingale Institute, Kings College (KCL) University of London, UK

Louise M. Long BSc (Hons), RGN, RM, DPSM, PGCEA
Lecturer in Midwifery, Nightingale Institute, King's College, University of London, UK

Maggie McNab MSc, RGN, RM, RHV
Primary Care Co-ordinator, West London Health Promotion Agency, London, UK

Val Thomas BA, MSc, RGN, RM
Project Director, Michigan Coalition on Substance Abuse Prevention, USA, formerly Health Promotion Co-ordinator, West London Health Promotion Agency, London, UK

Patricia Wilson MSc, RGN, RM
Former Parentcraft and Infant Feeding Sister, Hammersmith Hospital, London, UK

Foreword

The time around the birth of a baby represents the most critical opportunity for the improvement of health in human life. The perinatal period presents a window of opportunity, a sensitive time when the mother and family, with the good of their baby at heart, and feeling the need to review their own way of life, are generally committed to improving their own health and the health of their child.

Midwives, particularly given the strong role they are entitled to play in 'woman-centred services' are in a unique place to promote health, either directly or through the development of public health policy. Yet there is often a gap between policy and practice. Some midwives will be working in truly woman-centred services which allow them to practise to the full. Naturally, practising to the full entails effective health promotion. Other services will be further behind, and it may be more difficult to 'promote health' in such settings. Nevertheless, even in this situation, there is still much to be done. Health promotion, as Helen Crafter and the other authors of this book make clear, goes well beyond parentcraft classes and a little advice at antenatal visits. True health promotion is highly political, and entails an understanding of the social and political forces that influence our lives and well-being in a fundamental way. No responsible midwife can ignore, for example, the direct results of poverty or the need to be strategic in the promotion of health. In addition, the 'art and science' of health promotion requires clear frameworks, knowledge in its own right and a number of skills.

This book will be an essential tool to those midwives who wish to make the most of this most critical health opportunity of human life. It will help those midwives who wish to work with women in laying down a strong foundation for healthy, happy life and parenting, ensuring that our work has an impact not only on the present, but far into the future lives of mother, baby and family. In this way, midwives will play a crucial role in strengthening the foundations of our society. Edited by an experienced lecturer and practitioner, and written by a number of authors with strong expertise, *Health promotion in midwifery* is essential reading for any midwife who cares enough to help lay down this firm foundation for health.

Lesley Page
The Queen Charlotte's Professor of Midwifery Practice
The Centre for Midwifery Practice and Policy
The Wolfson School of Health Science
Thames Valley University
London, UK

Preface

Much of midwifery involves the art and science of health promotion. However the role of the midwife is observed, it soon becomes apparent that she spends the major part of her working days with generally healthy people (healthy enough, that is, to conceive and nurture a pregnancy), helping them to maintain their level of health, improve it and broaden it. The days of midwives 'doing antenatal checks', 'delivering babies' and 'checking the postpartum mother and baby' are surely numbered as midwives as a profession strive to improve the way that midwifery care is delivered by making it more appropriate to each woman's needs, and more evidence-based. The principles of general health promotion – good communication and information-sharing, understanding the basics of psychology, social and cultural issues, ethics and education (to name but a few), are important to the underpinning of good midwifery practice. This book attempts to bring together these concepts and many more specifically within the sphere of midwifery practice, using midwifery literature and research where applicable. However, just as no man is an island, so no profession works and evolves in isolation, and so information from complementary and allied academic fields is also applied where relevant, but very much with the role of the midwife in mind. The principles are addressed and the practice discussed because midwifery is and will always remain a very practical profession.

In laying the foundations of this book it has become apparent to me that there are enough literature and evidence in existence to develop theories of midwifery health promotion as a subset of the academic discipline of midwifery itself, and quite separate from the well-advanced studies in health promotion in nursing. Perhaps because of our very practical nature, we have been slow to develop our own frameworks and subdisciplines within the overall umbrella of midwifery.

Enough about midwives taking centre stage. In line with the current philosophy in the maternity services of 'woman-centred care', I am aware that my and my co-contributors' philosophies throughout this book are of individualized, woman- and family-centred care within the inescapable framework of bureaucracy, large organizations and sheer numbers of people. I am also aware that many midwives reading it will be acutely aware of the gap between this 'woman-centred' approach and the reality of what happens with the increasing use of more sophisticated technologies in obstetric care, where many of us find our practice is still to some extent dictated by policies, rules, protocols and the limited resources of time and money, especially in the hospital setting. Yet things are changing; who of us in practice would have thought ten, or even five years ago that the recommendations of the government reports into the maternity services chaired by Winterton and Cumberlege were even on the horizon, let alone being incorporated into required policy for health authorities?

For midwives who are well on the way to truly woman- and family-centred care, I hope this book helps you on your journey. For those still contemplating that difficult passage, or just embarking on a career as a midwife, I hope that this book will provide some of the strength and evidence that you need to commence your journey and dispense as far as possible with routine and out-of-date, hospital-centred practices. A balance is surely within our grasp for safe, practical midwifery and obstetric care which develops and empowers women.

As is usual in midwifery texts, the problem of reference to the midwife's gender cannot be accurately and concisely conveyed due to the limitations of English grammar. I have settled for 'she' and 'her' rather than the more clumsy 's/he', 'he/she' or 'her/his' but appreciate the problem this presents for some readers. My choice is because of the preponderance of women in midwifery, and in no way intends to demean the role that men play in the profession.

Every effort has been made to obtain copyright holders' permission where appropriate, but if material has been inadvertently overlooked the publishers will be happy to correct any oversights at the earliest opportunity.

Helen Crafter
London, 1997

Acknowledgements

I extend my heartfelt thanks to the following people who in a variety of ways offered me their time, wisdom, thoughts and experiences and made this book possible.

Alan Cribb and Jill Macleod Clark were extremely generous with their time and suggestions as my initial ideas came together. Brian Birch shared the agony and the ecstasy of being a writer at some early critical times and steered me towards some wonderfully inspiring texts about learning to *enjoy* writing. I name all my close work colleagues individually because their humour, ideas and encouragement have been a constant source of strength to me; Maureen Boyle, Huguette Comerasamy, Pauline Cooke, Christine Grabowska, Liz Hallewell, Sandra Macdonald, Julia Magill Cuerden, Merle Mullings, Lesley Page, Sue Scott, Caroline Squire, Gail Thomas, Nicola Winson and Margaret Yerby.

I feel I must particularly thank Damien Braganza in the Child Health Unit at OPCS (now the ONS) who on a number of occasions tracked down figures and statistics for me and was always extremely helpful and efficient.

Liz Floyd has been a wonderful friend to me over the years but her willingness to scrutinize and comment on an early draft of the book for me was more than any friend could reasonably expect. I am indebted to her for the care that she took, and the guidance she offered. Similarly my father has given up many hours to read and critique my work for little personal benefit other than to see the family name in print!

Jilly Rosser provided me with a great deal of inspiration as the book neared completion. My editors at Arnold, firstly Richard Holloway and latterly Fiona Goodgame and then Clare Parker, have been unfailing in their support and practical advice.

The women whose pregnancies and births I have been privileged to be involved in also deserve mention because they have shown me the light on many, many occasions. Similarly, the many student midwives and nurses I have met over the last few years, and midwives I have worked with as colleagues have shared ideas with me and helped me to formulate and develop my own thoughts and ideas.

Finally, a big thanks to my husband, Stephen Hine, who has only had half a wife, if that, for the last four years.

Helen Crafter
London, 1997

List of figures

Line figures

Photographs

List of tables

List of exercises

Part I

Principles

1

Health promotion and the midwife

Midwives are in an ideal position to extend support to expectant and new families and to provide a service which helps parents to access information and use it effectively to nurture the health of their family. However, they also have an important role in bringing to public attention those issues which are beyond the scope of individuals to change, such as social and environmental obstacles. These obstacles have major implications in undermining health and require community action in order to improve public health for everyone.

Health and birth

We all have our own ideas about what health is and isn't, although attempts have been made by experts over the years to produce a single meaning acceptable to everyone. The World Health Organization (WHO) for instance, since 1946, has offered 'a state of complete physical, mental and social well-being, and not merely the absence of disease or infirmity'. However the problem with such definitions is that they portray health as a quiescent condition, when in reality health for individuals is under constant challenge from the stresses and strains of daily living.

For health is indeed part of the struggle for survival by the most efficient means of adaptation that are available. Health may come easily to some fortunate people, but for many it requires a delicate combination of factors, some individual and some societal; it is also dependent for most of us on a hefty element of good luck. The struggle is both mental and physical, with strong environmental overtones. When adaptation to the constantly changing environment is not efficient, an optimal state of survival, i.e. health, can be compromised. So too with birth, which should be thought of in much the same dynamic terms, and the extreme effort which a woman necessarily invests in bringing a child into the world, is rewarded by conquest in the struggle against many odds – those of pain, disability and death, if indeed these odds are overcome.

Nowhere is the struggle for survival and health more apparent than at birth. For instance if the birth process is very long and the oxygen supply to the fetus becomes diminished, then more blood is automatically diverted to the brain and many metabolic defences come into play to prevent long-term fetal damage. Nature has made health a constant challenge, a contest to balance well-being and stave off ill-health. This contest rages within each one of us all of the time – fighting off infection, maintaining mental stability through stress and anxiety – and survival of the fittest is a reality in ensuring the continuation of our species through the healthiest in the population.

Unfortunately, survival of the human race as nature dictates makes individuals dispensable. Survival of the fittest makes for a more robust population but is careless of those who fall by the wayside and cannot compete by nature's strict, unwavering rules.

Medicine attempts to rewrite the laws of nature offering health (or as near as it can get) to a greater number of people, giving a helping hand in the struggle for survival. In this way the definition of health has come to be rewritten with different boundaries within which modern medicine can sometimes step to reinstate health where there is deficiency, particularly of a physical nature. However medicine is a powerful, enticing science which has not stopped at attempting to return people to health – nowadays, it attempts to improve on nature. Pain-free birth with an epidural anaesthetic, and decreased postpartum bleeding with the administration of a synthetic oxytocic drug are felt by many to improve on natural 'health' – although such interventions are not without their drawbacks and critics. Perhaps our greatest dilemma in promoting health generally, as in maternity care, is to know how to define and interpret normality, when to intervene in the process of childbearing and what the role of the health promoter should be.

The definition of health is a particularly complex one for midwives, many of whom work in an environment where pregnancy and birth are not seen as 'healthy' conditions (except perhaps in retrospect, when the 'danger' of birth has been overcome). To be in a state of 'complete . . . well-being' is hard enough to achieve for most people, but pregnancy and birth is a particular time in a woman's life noted for physical, mental and social changes, when the limits of 'normality' are exceptionally difficult to set.

If a midwife primarily sees her role as detecting and helping to correct ill-health or abnormality, she will be continually on the lookout for deviations from her predefined narrow outline of normality and, with extreme vigilance, will almost certainly find some. However if she sees childbirth as a normal physiological event, and believes that in most cases biological conditions are normal (or, if they are not, that they attempt to right themselves by a number of mechanisms with a minimum of outside interference) then she is likely to have a much broader concept of health. Yet in this second situation, her role will be quite different from that in the first; moving from a basically active diagnostic one to a supportive, more 'hands-off' role. Most midwives probably work somewhere in the middle of these two poles – intervening to help nature along rather than override it – and calling in help when things are not running smoothly, or when a medical opinion is felt to be required.

Through this confusion of meanings and boundaries of health and ill-health, the midwife must practise her profession. However, the confusion provides some clues as to why it is difficult for childbirth to be seen as a normal physiological event in the context of modern medicine, and why there are so many conflicting views and philosophies on how and where birth should take place in contemporary society. This book cannot provide all the answers and certainly cannot dictate a 'correct' philosophy, but without a genuine respect for health and nature, and the birth process in the context of the struggle to achieve health, it will prove difficult for the practising midwife of the future to be clear about how the increasing sophistication of health technology can fit in with the respect and individual attention which, as a basic human right, must be extended to all childbearing women and their families.

What is health promotion?

The concept of health promotion has emerged with the increasing realization in society that health can and should be improved for many people, and that our health is one of our most valuable personal assets.

There is also increasing evidence that in reality individuals have limited control over their own well-being. Although people obviously do hold some responsibility and should be given free choice to behave as they wish (as long as their action does not harm others), considerations such as a balanced diet, a sound mental constitution and a decision not to smoke or abuse drugs are influenced by many factors that are beyond individual control. The financial means to buy nutritious food, the ability to manage one's finances, having a stable and supportive family and living in an environment where it is the exception rather than the norm to smoke, and where self-esteem is high enough to resist temptations that may lead a person to take an apparent short cut to escaping the drudgeries in life, will strongly influence the health 'choices' that people make.

Health promotion therefore acknowledges the role of the community in fostering awareness, social support and the autonomy and empowerment of its members, as well as making health accessible to all. These are seen as crucial if health and welfare are to be improved in all of society's members, including (and most importantly) those who are least able to access information and actively seek 'good health' – the poor, the non-English speakers and everyone for whom having control over their lives seems to be the terrain of the articulate middle classes or well-organized pressure groups.

Health promotion is an activity requiring the participation of all 'stakeholders' in order to be successful. Where, for instance, an improvement in the health of pregnant women in an inner city estate is considered, the opinions and knowledge of the women themselves are vital if strategies are to be developed that are sensitive to the circumstances in which the women and their families live. Such a policy designed and implemented by policymakers and health professionals without such community involvement is destined to failure because the women will have things done to them by outsiders, rather than having their real needs respected and valued. If such women do not have a stake in the aims and implementation of a project or care scheme, then any benefits that are seen are unlikely to be sustained. Health promotion therefore incorporates understanding and responding to people's needs, rather than anticipating those needs and their answers. The same is true of health promotion activities undertaken by an individual midwife dealing with individual women; exploration with each woman of her knowledge and opinions, and respect of them is crucial if the woman is to feel that her midwifery care is of value to her.

Health promotion can only be effective if it is understood that health depends on a multitude of factors which have complicated and, as yet, poorly understood interrelations. The most apparent of these factors include people's values, attitudes and behaviour, and the relationship between them; people's self-esteem and personality; their social environment and employment status; the quality of housing and family relationships. It is not essential (and probably not possible) for the health promoter to understand the relationship in individuals between their personality, housing status and health for instance, but it is necessary to be aware that a relationship exists, and that health is manipulated by circumstances that are neither simple nor swift to change.

A major challenge for health promotion concerns the existence of environmental pollutants whose growth in industry remains largely unchecked, and which may be responsible for some congenital abnormalities and chronic health problems. There is relatively little information circulated in public about the chemicals discharged into our water supplies, the drugs, pesticides and questionable foodstuffs fed to animals destined to enter the human food chain, and nuclear power and waste disposal, except that which is circulated (and usually funded) by the industries themselves. Such issues often only receive widespread public attention when crises such as Creutzfeldt–Jakob disease, or leukaemia clusters around nuclear plants become newsworthy items. These and other issues are slowly but increasingly being aired through non-government funded public campaigns, yet this is a good example of where individuals have very limited control over the way such environmental problems may affect them and where structured, community-based health promotion, often in the form of pressure groups, is more able to raise public awareness.

However, in defining what health promotion is, it becomes important to acknowledge some of the misunderstanding about health promotion in society, particularly what control individuals have over their own health. The Research Unit in Health and Behavioural Change in Edinburgh (1989) commented that there is a traditional view in society, still widely held, that individual behaviour is both the prime cause of ill-health, and a major factor in the maintenance and attainment of good health. Like many other researchers and authors (for instance Townsend and Davidson, 1988; Jacobson *et al.*, 1991), the Research Unit demonstrate effectively how this is not the case, and that individuals have remarkably little control over their health status. But if this is what many people believe, how have such beliefs come about? The answer partly lies in the rise and success of medical ideology, which values highly the expert knowledge of health professionals, especially doctors. It woos society, particularly through the media, into expectations of excellent cure rates and eradication of infectious diseases and other medical disorders. People want to believe that life is relatively safe, and if they or loved ones fall ill, then they can be saved. However, putting all one's faith into one solution has many problems, and if the health professions cannot prevent or cure ill-health, then in order for the public to maintain their faith, a let-out clause for medical 'failures' must be found. An apparently easily believable rationale is that if individuals can be blamed for their failing health in the first place (for smoking perhaps, or not eating 'healthy' food), then medicine cannot be blamed for ineffectiveness. The problem with such 'victim blaming' is that the wrongs of society are conveniently excused, and the need to address the socio-economic and environmental issues is avoided. However without addressing these complicated attitudes and beliefs, it is difficult to imagine how the long-term health of society can be improved in any significant, sustainable way.

There is therefore some confusion at present about what health promotion is, sometimes because a health professional will label an activity 'health promotion' when it patently is not. An example may be a parent education class on infant feeding where both the topic and the content of the session are decided by the midwife. Although safe infant feeding is closely associated with health, and a midwife expounding the virtues of breastfeeding and hygiene in making up formula feed may be seen by the midwife involved as 'promoting health', such a teaching style is not commensurate with the effective improvement of health. There may be some gains in increased understanding if the midwife happens to have anticipated some of her audience's needs, but if attitudes are not explored and challenged, and individual social contexts of the participants not acknowledged, benefit will be limited.

There is a temptation to label any activity that addresses health issues, however poorly, 'health promotion' because the term is in vogue. It is also much easier to decide what people need rather than to ask them, and start the painstaking process of listening, questioning one's own values and beliefs and sharing power and releasing control, which true health promotion necessarily involves. It may be awesome for individual midwives to consider such an approach, especially if they personally value modern medicine uncritically.

In promoting health it is important for the midwife to recognize her limitations, as well as utilizing her personal and professional strengths. Her role in the health of the nation's new families can be small but significant for the families she supports; but it will be small and insignificant if she has not targeted the needy with good support and listening skills, and taken an active interest in attempting to understand the complicated issues that surround the political aspects of health and its distribution in society.

Health promotion and health education

The terms 'health promotion' and 'health education' are often used interchangeably, but it is important to be aware that there are differences in meaning between the two.

Health promotion is a more recent description of the work done by such professionals as midwives, nurses, doctors, teachers, health promotion officers and others in broadly moving the population towards better health, often by addressing health policy through collective action as we have seen, but also in considering the influences on people's health other than those which can be addressed through education. Health education up to the mid-1980s focused on individual and group learning, dealing with themes such as a good diet and a wise lifestyle as the way to well-being. The idea of health promotion, on the other hand, has developed as more extensive issues such as environmental hazards and health inequalities have surfaced in public awareness. As there is so little that private individuals or non-political groups can do about such issues, solutions to problems will come only as public attitudes are developed. Whereas health education encompasses the provision and sharing of information and changing attitudes and behaviour (jobs which the midwife is ideally placed to do), health promotion also involves marshalling societal, governmental and indeed global responsibility for the health of individuals and communities.

A further difference suggested by French (1985) is that health promotion is seen by many as a more scientific activity than health education, being more amenable to quantitative evaluation. It is easier to measure changes in the health of a community, for instance by setting targets as in *The health of the nation* (Department of Health, 1992) with such markers as teenage pregnancy rates or general population smoking rates, than it is to measure the quality of information provided in leaflets, or changes in attitudes or behaviour. However, greater ease of measuring outcomes does not necessarily make an activity better; it is just easier to justify its financial and work outlay. The success or otherwise of health promotion is no doubt partly due to the groundwork of the professionals who take the time and care to listen to individuals and groups, while being aware of the broader issues which may militate against immediate shifts in attitude or behaviour, or against health itself.

The term health education will be used in this book to refer to education in its true liberal sense, of responding to individuals and small groups who wish to gain and share better knowledge and understanding of their health. Health promotion is used as a broader term, particularly to refer to the very wide range of activities that are pursued to achieve better health, and the policy and action required to make better health attainable for more people.

Midwives' personal concepts of health

It is important for us as midwives to consider our own concepts of health, both in relation to our own well-being and that of others, because this affects the way we offer, deliver and evaluate care for women and families. For instance, a midwife who smokes yet is expected as part of her role to encourage discontinuation of smoking in childbearing women, will be influenced in the way she gives care in different ways from a non-smoking midwife, partly because of her own lifestyle. Similarly, midwives may or may not themselves be mothers and this experience again will affect the way professional care is perceived and given. Greater insight into our own beliefs and behaviour can only enhance the quality of care we are able to give. This is not to say that midwives who smoke or have not experienced pregnancy and motherhood give less good care – indeed, their experiences may be used to achieve greater insight – but all of us benefit from reflecting on why we believe what we believe in relation to health and birth, and relating this to our practice.

We interpret other women's experiences of childbirth through our own values and beliefs. Consider the following hypothetical case histories, those of Lucy and Grace. Are both of them healthy, or is one or are both of them in less than optimal health? Who knows better, Lucy or her doctor, or you or Grace? Can two people have different answers, and both be right? These questions are difficult to answer, yet impossible for today's midwife to ignore.

> Lucy, 28, has been confined to a wheelchair since her late teens following a road traffic accident. She is relatively independent at home, but relies on her husband Bob for help with aspects of daily living outside their home. Although medically advised not to have a child by her doctor, who feels she is not independent enough to cope with the day-to-day care of a baby while Bob is out at work, Lucy has considered her abilities carefully and she and Bob feel that, with his full cooperation, she will be able to manage. They embark on a pregnancy.

> Grace is 45 years old and smokes thirty cigarettes a day. She has no symptoms from her 30-year-old habit apart from a productive cough which she has had for 10 years. She is pregnant.

Applying the WHO definition of health to such women clearly has limitations. For instance, Lucy's GP has no experience of her day-to-day physical abilities and limitations, and may have no experience of physical handicap other than on a professional basis, seeing and speaking with patients only when they have difficulties which lead them to consult with their doctor. Grace may sail through her pregnancy and produce a large healthy baby at the end of it; or she may develop haemoptysis or a thrombosis, which may or may not compromise her health in the long term. The definition takes no account of individuals like Lucy and Grace and their long-term situations, or how they feel and cope on a day-to-day basis.

Health and, for that matter, illness tend nowadays to be described as a changing, dynamic continuum of 'physical, psychological [emotional, cognitive and developmental] spiritual and social components and adaptive behavioural responses to internal and external stimuli' (Murray and Zentner, 1989:5). Health is not seen in this definition as a static condition, and although the challenge of resisting ill-health can be seen as a positive move, the ideal of the WHO description of health has been replaced with a more realistic and careful balance of adaptive behaviours and responses. Also, for each individual, society takes a role in determining health; one's family, friends, job and general environment all play a part.

This idea of holism has taken on more importance in recent years. Dines and Cribb (1993) describe a number of elements concerned with holism, including the concepts of people as a 'whole' and society as a 'whole'. The general idea is that in categorizing individuals or societies, using labels indicating, say, levels of physical or psychological well-being, vital clues are missed where there is a linkage or interaction between categories, as for example between being in a state of depression and being unemployed. This is especially true for a woman at the time of her giving birth, when it is considered necessary in giving good care to see the woman not just as a human incubator for her child but also as an individual with a life, perhaps as a homeless person, a company director, a refugee, a happily single woman or a newly deserted wife. Situations in which women find themselves when newly pregnant are as individual as the women themselves, and pregnancy is as much a psychological process as it is a physical one. As we look at a woman holistically, her family, friends and environment will all play their part in defining her experience as a mother.

Reflection on personal concepts of health will no doubt reveal internal conflicts for many of us. Home birth with a first baby is a good example; while some midwives will feel that this is a safe option for the majority of women, many midwives will feel that it is definitely not the safest option. Many of us probably now feel that we lack the experience of home birth to form a strong opinion on its safety, although opinions are often much easier to come by than factual evidence! Yet women's experiences of birth are known to be crucial to their mental well-being, and place of birth must surely be an important factor of this state of mental health. Chapter 2 contains an exercise through which you can reflect on your own ideas about what health is, how health and illness are experienced and expressed, and how these ideas and concepts may be rooted in childhood, where many influences play a part.

Because they work in the public domain, midwives must take account of other people's concepts of health in forming their own, and be accepting of other people who do not necessarily share their values and ideas. The easiest way to find out how another person feels about issues such as health, pregnancy and childrearing is to ask her, but there are also studies being continually done and reported in the professional literature, which compare and contrast lay views of health. Such studies come up with general themes which can be applied to practice where a midwife feels this is appropriate. Such a study is described in Chapter 11 by Pat Wilson, who explores with women their understanding of health in pregnancy, and their reaction to the health advice they have been given. A further example of such a study (Crawford, 1993) analyses interviews with sixty adults in the United States, asking them 'Are you healthy? How do you know?' Although not a British sample, and not one of pregnant women, the author's emerging themes will seem familiar to many midwives as perhaps applicable to many adults in the Western world. They commonly included self-control and discipline, self-denial, willpower, self-blame and self-responsibility. In considering why personal responsibility is such a strong thread in these interviews, Crawford suggests that health promotion should be understood in the context of culture. He concludes, 'The body and "personal responsibility" for health is, I believe, the symbolic terrain upon which both the desire for control and the display of control are exacted' (p. 138). In Western cultures, control of our personal lives is an important issue and significant measures of that control are our health, fitness, longevity and ability to have children at a time when we so choose.

Styles of health promotion – moving from the traditional to the radical

All too often health professionals can still be found who seem to expect people to do exactly as they are told. Such a style of 'health promotion' – although it is now clear that this is not health promotion, or even health education – is ineffective because people do not simply do what they are told is good for them. If they did, no one would smoke, abuse alcohol or take drugs and practically all babies would be breastfed. Yet this style of 'health promotion' has been around for a long time, and has traditionally largely been about attempting to get people to change their behaviour by persuasion, occasionally coercion, and latterly a very narrow view of education. But if this way of trying to improve health is so ineffective, why is it still in existence? There are probably a number of reasons. First, it is easier than the alternatives. Caught in the middle of a busy antenatal clinic with many 'bookings' to complete, it is far less time consuming to give a woman a 'lecture' about the benefits of breastfeeding than to spend time exploring with her how she feels about it, and building on what she thinks the advantages and disadvantages for her are. Some midwives may not feel that they are doing their job properly if they do not stress what is 'best' for the baby. It may then seem easy to escape responsibility if the woman does not take such advice – a midwife may describe this as the woman's choice and blame her for a poor decision. It may also be easier for health professionals to slip into the role of traditional 'health promotion' because lay people have a generally uncritical acceptance of the belief that 'doctor (or health professional) knows best' – and it can feel more comfortable to feel valued and respected for one's professional knowledge, especially if self-confidence is not high.

Radical styles of health promotion are by no means easier to effect, because midwives at present continue to practise in an environment where medical culture is strong. However, more radical styles of health promotion must move away from concentrating on the individual to studying individuals in the context of their environment. Although such a re-think should lead to a more holistic approach to promoting health, this can only occur if a critical approach is fostered, which not only rejects the traditional belief that medical expertise in normal pregnancy and birth must take precedence over what women want for themselves, but acknowledges the insidious effect on the way both lay people and health professionals think and behave. A political awareness of health issues is also paramount to prevent an attempted move to more radical health promotion becoming little more than rhetoric.

A shift away from traditional 'health promotion' requires us to question previous practice, formulate new health policy, re-educate professionals and embark on new research which reflects real needs in society. Such a shift is not easy but radical health promotion in recent times has led to a greater amount of maternity care taking place in the community, the questioning of induction of labour and Caesarean section rates, and a critical analysis of fetal screening tests with calls for more research into the long-term emotional consequences for women of undergoing such investigations.

Who needs health promotion?

The meaning of 'need' is an interesting point where health promotion is concerned, because humanity has managed to survive until now without health being particularly promoted. In Britain, structured health promotion in the form of public health probably dates from Victorian times, when sanitary measures such as cleaning up water supplies were effected to control the deadly spread of diseases such as typhoid and cholera. However, in the last 50 years or so there has been a further growth in the popular understanding that general standards of health can and should be improved. This has occurred against a background of arguments about the 'bottomless pit' of social needs, with problems in deciding where the money necessary to make improvements should come from. The National Health Service makes insatiable demands on the public purse, and health promotional activities are only one aspect of its work. Therefore it is necessary to assess need in some way, and measure outcomes of success. The evaluation of health promotion will be addressed in a future chapter, but prior to this, midwives need to consider how they assess the needs of individuals and societies, and whether their assessment is fair and rational.

A need occurs when a set of circumstances requires a course of action. In 1972, Jonathan Bradshaw attempted the difficult task of attempting to break down the concept of social need into more measurable units in order to assess requirements more rationally than can be done without such a quantifiable framework. In his now classic and frequently quoted work he writes of

- *normative need* – a desirable standard laid down by the professional, often in the form of a set of rules or a policy manual;
- *felt need* – or what people actually want. This is the most nebulous of Bradshaw's needs and may eventually become an
- *expressed need* – that is, the service demanded by an individual or a group of people; and
- *comparative need* – which occurs where the recipients of a service are compared to assess gaps and inequality in provision. The need is to bring about equality and fairness.

These concepts are clearly useful in assessing health needs, by making them more definable and less abstract. For instance, in understanding that a felt need may not automatically lead to an expressed need because of lack of opportunity, information or motivation, a midwife may become sensitive to a woman's need to formulate and vocalize her ideas, thereby increasing her confidence and the quality of her birth experience. Exercise 1.1 is designed to enable you to apply types of need in practice.

Both individuals and societies are required to make decisions about whether specific circumstances require action, in health matters as well as in other concerns. Where some governments will elect not to take action where a health need is not perceived to be great enough, another government may have acted much earlier. Also in the same society, the governing body may modify its policy over time, perceiving a need where previously it felt none; or vice versa, perceiving that a health need has disappeared and action is no longer required.

There will never be universal agreement on health needs because health does not and cannot command a universal consensus of opinion. The issues of tobacco advertising and the role of the welfare state in improving health are examples of political hot potatoes, where a multitude of opinions and policies conflict in both their values and underlying philosophies. However, collectives, often an elected local or central government, will usually give guidelines (decided by economy, policy and ethic) as to the limits of support it will give to individuals in fulfilling their own needs, and to agents (e.g. health promoters) to offer fulfilment of need to consumers.

A good example of a health need which is being explored in the field of midwifery is that of continuity of carer for women through pregnancy, birth and the early puerperium. A number of studies (for instance Davies and Evans, 1991; Hutton, 1994; Oakley, 1996) have expressed the need felt over a number of years, of women from all sections of society (including midwives and, in the case of Ann Oakley's team, social scientists), for

---

EXERCISE 1.1   The concept of social need

1.   Normative need
How are the normative needs of women formalized in your work setting? (If there is a 'Standard Setting' or 'Clinical Quality Assurance' team in your place of work they will have details.) What normative needs have been formally accepted by your organization?

2.   Felt need
Reflect on the care you have recently offered to a pregnant or labouring woman. Did you perceive any felt needs which she had, through your intuition? Because women in well-established labour are often unable to communicate through words and meaningful dialogue, this is an important and sensitive element of practice for midwives. How have you personally dealt with your perception of her felt need?

3.   Expressed need
Which voluntary organizations do you perceive as most vocal in demanding changes in health provision for maternity care and young families? Have they made any difference in the service provision you see around you?

4.   Comparative need
Do the women you observe accessing maternity care receive comparative care? What general and individual factors affect comparable care, or prevent its deliverance? If you have access to information about another maternity unit, do women have comparable access to, for instance, fetal screening tests?

---

more continuity of care from a midwife, or small group of midwives, primarily appointed to give such attention. In the early 1990s the Government in office appointed one of its Members of Parliament, Nicholas Winterton, to explore this expressed need and report on its significance in contemporary society (Health Committee Second Report, 1991–92). Winterton, in his summing up of the evidence which he received from many sources, indeed confirmed that not only was this need strongly felt, but that it was time to take action in the form of an Expert Group being set up to advise on future maternity policy and practice. The need for continuity of care and carer, among other recommendations, became normative – that is, a standard needed to be set, whereby the maternity service providers and users knew of a basic minimum standard required for providing and receiving continuity of care in an environment of more 'woman-centred' care.

So much for the needs of populations which, although not always met, are often widely expressed through pressure groups set up with a specific purpose in mind. There is a need to be wary of overt statements of health need because they are almost always made by the articulate, who are able to shout the loudest. It is more useful for the midwife to assess individual health needs against a background of knowledge of her own political awareness – that of the effects of poverty, poor housing, problems in speaking and understanding the English language, marital violence and endemic racism. Although she will not be able to solve the inadequacies of society overnight, her understanding will provide her with a much more effective background in really understanding the greatest needs of the women in her care.

Local data can be used for assessing the needs of childbearing women. Maternity units are required to keep figures on, for instance, Caesarean and instrumental delivery rates, induction of labour and mortality and morbidity statistics. These are often collated for all Health Authorities in Annual Health Reports, but many units also now audit their own figures as a form of quality control. Such statistics may be used for planning service provision as well as for evaluating the quality of the service.

However, just as health is not a state that can be measured with precision, nor are health needs straightforward. In assessing such needs, the midwife will be influenced by her own knowledge, attitudes and prejudices; life and professional experience and intuition; the environment culture and organization in which she works, and to some extent by how fulfilled her own needs are. In few other fields is it so important for the needs of people to be accurately and sensitively assessed, as it is in those of childbearing women and their families.

EXERCISE 1.2   Reflective exercise

How do you anticipate women's needs? Why do you spend more time with some women than others? Is it always because of the woman's need, or are there other factors to do with you or the organization in which you work?

Women's health promotion and health messages portrayed in the media

The targeting of specific groups for health promotion, such as the sexually active, women or smokers, has become increasingly popular over recent years. It is not difficult to see why this has come about – gathering together an apparently homogeneous group can make health promotional activities more relevant and more tailored to suit selected candidates.

Women's health, often addressed in the clinical field in the form of well women's clinics, family planning clinics and menopause clinics, requires critical debate as well as practical application. Political issues such as equality between the sexes, affordable childcare for women wishing to study and work outside the home, and poverty as it affects women are often ignored in health care issues such as providing suitable contraception, dealing with violence against women within the home and preventing women's cancers. One of the criticisms of targeting women for health care is that health education programmes for women have traditionally focused on women's health problems and needs in the context of assumed traditional roles as mothers and carers, thereby perpetuating the idea that women are primarily responsible for family health and wellbeing. Although this may well be the reality of what happens in many families, health promotion could be accused of furthering the great burden put upon women not only of being expected to work outside the home, but also of continuing to hold most of the responsibility for organizing what goes on within it. If a mother is both a wage earner (as the majority of women are) and also the primary homemaker, it is difficult to see how equality of the sexes can be realized. The continuing dominance of men over women in the Western world, as demonstrated by the imbalance of the sexes in politics, boardrooms and public schools, further illustrates the difficulties for the promoter of women's health in deciding how much of her practice should reinforce contemporary cultural, social and health issues, and how much it should challenge them.

The difficulties of knowing how best to deal with women's health issues are compounded by the way that health messages directed at women are portrayed in the media. These messages are frequently formulated by the attitudes of those sending them towards women, and these are all too often male, middle-class news editors. Furthermore the 'evidence' that is known about women's health has been subverted by medical, political and commercial interests. Parrott and Condit (1996), in their evaluation of the way that women's health messages influence contemporary health issues, also suggest that health care is often depicted by the media as a science, thereby offering knowledge and clear answers. This is compounded when a doctor is interviewed (giving the message that he or she is an expert), and asked to explain an issue in a few sentences, which are then broadcast or printed as 'fact' (or at least little or no time is given to an alternative viewpoint). The public are then generally left with the impression that health issues are simple and the same for everyone.

What then should be the role of health promotion directed at women? It is not good enough for it to formulate simple, unsophisticated aims which ignore the social and economic conditions in which women live, or base its aims on the social and economic conditions of men and assume that women share these. Amos (1993) suggests that it should empower women by addressing the structural factors which shape women's lives and health opportunities, and avoid reinforcing gender stereotypes and social inequalities by emphasizing individual solutions for the ills of society. It is therefore not appropriate for a midwife to teach a woman about eating a healthy diet in pregnancy without checking that the diet suggested is culturally acceptable and that any proposed foods are affordable. Mid-wives have a further professional responsibility in bringing to the attention of society the difficulties inherent in pregnancy and early parenthood as a result of poverty, poor social conditions and gender and culture stereotyping.

The goals of health promotion

Goals or aims in an activity such as health promotion are important because they indicate to everyone what the activity expects to achieve. They are also important because they allow evaluation to take place by measuring what occurs against what the health promoter wanted to occur for the activity to be considered a success. (Evaluating health promotion activities will be explored in Chapter 7.)

Goals usually pivot around the themes of process and product. The 'process' of health promotion involves the way in which people gain information and understanding, and how their decision-making skills are enhanced in using the information (or disregarding it as they see fit). The process of health promotion, even when goals are specific, is notoriously difficult to measure. The 'product' of health promotion, or the end result, is often quantifiable and therefore more easy to measure, but large numbers of people may be required to make the result statistically significant, and the multitude of other factors that may lead to such a result may not be taken into account.

As an illustration of formulating goals of a health promotion activity, teenage sex education is a good example. In terms of process, the health promoter may decide that their goals are to raise awareness of sexual issues among teenagers, and provide a forum where relationships, personal values and contraceptive methods can be openly discussed and explored. The product goal following such an activity may be to reduce the teenage unwanted pregnancy rate.

Goals of health promotion should reflect the needs of the participants, not those of the health promoter. In raising awareness of sexual issues with teenagers, some of them may choose to plan their pregnancies in seemingly dire social circumstances (although it could be argued that this is about poor educational opportunity and socio-economic factors rather than true choice). It may be unpalatable to accept individuals' decisions about their lives, but this does not allow health promoters to decide what is best for other people.

Many of the issues in this scenario are best dealt with at community level rather than with individuals; to reduce the overall teenage unwanted pregnancy rate, national policy is required to address the issues of education and socio-economic problems which affect young people. The issues should also be defined by teenagers themselves; they best know the pressures, problems and realities in their lives, and they hold the key to how these areas can best be addressed. The work of grassroots health promoters has relatively little impact on the deep-seated reasons as to why teenage unwanted pregnancy rates are so high in the UK, despite sex education being taught in the school curriculum. A reduction in the rate is only likely to be achieved if national as well as local decisions are made about both the 'process' and 'product' goals of health promotion.

Summary of key points

- Health means different things to different people. It incorporates a delicate combination of factors, some individual and some societal. Adequate definitions of health, like birth, should incorporate cultural and environmental overtones. If birth is not seen as a normal, cultural and/or family-centred event, this has negative implications for the role and responsibilities of the midwife as a health promoter.
- Health is one of our most valuable personal assets. It can be improved for many people, particularly the increasing numbers of people living in poverty, of which women and children are particularly at risk.
- While health education is an effective form of health promotion if the needs of participants are explored, it is a small part of the broader, more politically aware picture of health promotion.
- The focus for improving public health must be on social policy which is sensitive to the needs and circumstances of all groups in society, not just the most vocal. To be effective, health professionals must work with people as participants, not recipients.
- Health promotion must acknowledge the complicated inter-relationships between socio-economic and environmental factors, and health. Individual behaviour is not the ultimate cause of ill-health, and therefore the general health of society will not be greatly improved by health promotion being specifically targeted at individuals.
- It is useful for the midwife to be aware of the theory of social need, and to develop her own theory of how her practice can most effectively promote health.
- The ultimate aim of health promotion (in line with its philosophy of the individual right to self-determination) is that people develop

control in their lives that enables them to choose if they so wish, and as freely as possible, the healthiest option that suits their particular circumstances. However, political policymakers may also state more quantifiable targets that may not be entirely consistent with self-determination.
* The field of women's health has been subverted by medical, political and commercial interests. Midwives should be careful not to perpetuate gender and cultural stereotypes of women when they provide health care, and be critically aware of the implications of what has previously been considered 'routine' practice.

References

Amos, A. 1993: In her own best interests? Women and health education: a review of the last fifty years. *Health Education Journal* 52(3), 141–50.

Bradshaw, J. 1972: The concept of social need. *New Society* 19, 640–3.

Crawford, R. 1993: A cultural account of 'health': Control, release and the social body. In Beattie, A., Gott, M., Jones, L. and Siddell, M. (eds), *Health and wellbeing: a reader*. Basingstoke: Macmillan in association with The Open University, 133–43.

Davis, J. and Evans, F. 1991: The Newcastle Community Midwifery Care Project. In Robinson, S. and Thompson, A.E. (eds), *Midwives, research and childbirth* Vol. 2. London: Chapman and Hall, 104–39.

Department of Health 1992: *The health of the nation*. London: HMSO.

Dines, A. and Cribb, A. 1993: *Health promotion concepts and practice*. Oxford: Blackwell Scientific.

French, J. 1985: To educate or promote health? *Health Education Journal* 44(3), 115–16.

Health Committee Second Report, Session 1991–92: *Maternity services*. London: HMSO.

Hutton E. 1994: What women want from midwives. *British Journal of Midwifery* 2(12), 608–11.

Jacobson, B., Smith, A. and Whitehead, M. (eds) 1991: *The nation's health: a strategy for the 1990's*. London: King's Fund Centre.

Murray, R.B. and Zentner J.P. 1989: *Nursing concepts for health promotion*. Hemel Hempstead: Prentice Hall.

Oakley, A. 1996: Social Support in pregnancy: does it have long-term effects? *Journal of Infant and Reproductive Psychology* 14, 7–22.

Parrott, R.L. and Condit, M.C. 1996: *Evaluating women's health messages*. Thousand Oaks, USA: Sage.

Research Unit in Health and Behavioural Change 1989: *Changing the public health*. Chichester: John Wiley and Sons.

Townsend, P. and Davidson, N. 1988: The Black Report. In *Inequalities in health*. Harmondsworth: Penguin, 29–213.

World Health Organization (WHO) 1946: *Constitution*. New York: WHO.

Further reading

Blaxter, M. 1990: *Health and lifestyles*. London: Routledge.

Ewles, L. and Simnett, I. 1995: *Promoting health: a practical guide*. London: Scutari Press.

Rodmell, S. and Watt, A. (eds) 1986: *The politics of health education*. London: Routledge and Kegan Paul.

Seedhouse, D. 1986: *Health: the foundations for achievement*. Chichester: John Wiley and Sons.

Tones, K. and Tilford, S. 1994: *Health education: effectiveness, efficiency and equity*. London: Chapman and Hall.

2

Personal and cultural influences on health

Having looked in the previous chapter at the meaning of health with particular reference to childbearing, and some preliminary ideas about what makes a midwife effective in her role in enhancing health, this chapter will look at the issues of early influences on the health of individuals, particularly their personal and family circumstances and the effect of cultural pressures and general education. In drawing on perspectives from other professional fields such as psychology and sociology, a broadening perspective of the midwife's role in health promotion will be developed.

The development of personality

Our personality is crucial to the way we interpret and react to health and ill-health, childbirth and parenthood. Like defining health, deciding what we mean by 'personality' also has its problems in that a simple, adequate definition does not exist. Psychologists refer to recurring characteristics and patterns of behaviour in a person, which demonstrate their interests, attitudes and abilities and suggest a reasonably constant reaction to the environment.

Personality is formed primarily within early family life. It has genetic, social and environmental elements, all of which combine to generate a unique person. Personality theories, developed mainly in the field of psychology, can help us to understand some aspects of people's characters but because the nature of personality is so wide the theories can only give us limited insights into what makes us the way we are. Also it should be remembered that such theories are developed over time and are subject to change, development and even rejection.

Some of the most famous personality theories were developed by Sigmund Freud (1856–1939), an Austrian physician and founding father of psychoanalysis, who described the underlying personality structures as the id (unconscious inherited processes), the ego (the guard of the id; requiring behaviour acceptable to the outside world), and the super ego (from which the conscience develops). Freud also described defence mechanisms, which allow the individual to protect his or her ego and super ego from conflicts which threaten the status quo of existence. His examples of defence mechanisms include denial, repression and sublimation. Freud believed that these processes generally went on in the subconscious with only occasional forays into the conscious, and influenced all of our day-to-day thoughts and human interactions. His theories are popular partly because his ideas can be explained simply and followed easily when we observe the way people react in different situations.

More recently, the psychologist Abraham Maslow developed a 'Hierarchy of needs' (Figure 2.1), which encapsulates the development of personality from birth to adulthood, based on the philosophy that in normal circumstances people are motivated, or moved to achieve more and more sophisticated needs in order to find self-fulfilment and 'self-actualization' – the feeling of being comfortable with oneself.

Maslow's hierarchy is often used to demonstrate the stepping stones in life's developmental processes, and midwives will recognize many of the stages mirrored in pregnancy, childbirth and early motherhood; for instance, esteem needs can be met when a woman feels she has achieved her goals of the birth (be it safe delivery, or perhaps birth with optimal drug usage) or self-fulfilment in reaching her potential. For some women, giving birth and becoming a mother will be their ultimate life experience, described by many as the most important, significant event of their life. Perhaps at this point we should ask ourselves, how important midwives are in helping women along the stepping stones of the hierarchy towards 'self-actualization' in the professional care that they give. Certainly, midwives have a major input in some of Maslow's stages – offering safe care, accepting women and families for what they are as they present themselves to the maternity services, and enhancing women's self-esteem by helping them to explore and understand their experiences.

There are many important writers on the subject of personality and personal development, and one of the most important twentieth-century psychologists is Carl Rogers, who introduces two central features into his theories of personality; those of self-concept and positive regard.

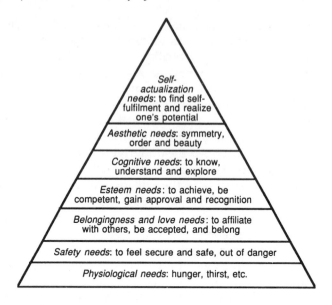

Figure 2.1 'Maslow's hierarchy of needs'. From *Motivation and personality,* 3rd edn by Abraham H. Maslow. Revised by Robert Frager *et al.* Copyright © 1954, 1987 by Harper & Row, Publishers, Inc. Copyright © 1970 by Abraham H. Maslow. Reprinted by permission of Addison-Wesley Educational Publishers Inc.

Self-concept depends on how an individual sees himself or herself in the world; how this affects his or her behaviour, and how that individual views the world. Rogers' ideal self-concept is positive regard. Internal anxiety is evoked, he believes, when the individual does not behave or perform in the way expected, and self-esteem is reduced when the self-concept conflicts with behaviour.

It is only possible here to brush over a few of the theories of personality development that exist, but even so they serve to illustrate the importance and relevance to midwifery of a basic knowledge of such explanations. Some of the titles listed in further reading at the end of this chapter include detail about personality theory.

However personality develops, there is widespread agreement that its primary, most fundamental influence is the family, in whatever form this takes. It is within the social context of the family that health and ill-health occur and are witnessed by impressionable young children. They are exposed to their parents' (or guardians') ideas of health, nutrition, exercise and so forth, and observe their parents' reactions to illness, childbirth and disability. Parents' beliefs and values are an important pattern for children's developing ideas, and present a 'norm' against which the new ideas of outsiders can be tested and considered. Exercise 2.1 may help you to reflect on the way you have come to think about health and ill-health.

EXERCISE 2.1   The influence of family on health

This exercise is designed to encourage you to reflect on some of your basic, early beliefs about health. You may wish also to consider whether and how these beliefs influence your professional behaviour.

Think back to your own childhood.

(a)   How did your family maintain your health?
(b)   What attitudes/roles did members of your family take when someone was ill?
(c)   When you were a youngster, how did your family deal with the issues of smoking, alcohol consumption, drug abuse and sex education?
(d)   How do you think your early experiences influence your attitudes to your own and friends' illnesses?
(e)   If you have ever discussed childbirth with your mother (or a close female relative), do you think her attitudes to and experiences of birth colour your own at all? If so, in what ways?

The desire to breastfeed is a good example of family-held values. A daughter is much more likely to breastfeed her own child if she herself was breastfed (Sloper *et al.*, 1975) because for her it will be the normal way to nourish her infant. The confidence of likely success is also transmitted from mother to daughter. Breastfeeding is also a good example of a pattern of health behaviour for which personal and cultural influences are strong. O'Campo *et al.* (1992) discovered that of all the psychosocial and demographic factors examined in their research into breastfeeding duration, four of the most important influences were normative beliefs, maternal confidence, social learning and behavioural beliefs about breastfeeding. This is not to say that there are not many other factors which motivate women to breastfeed, such as information provided by other women and health professionals during pregnancy (see Chapter 14), but such information is sometimes rejected by a new mother if it is contrary to the values she absorbed in the earlier part of her life. Aspects of her personality such as flexibility and degree of openness to new ideas will influence her reaction to alternative beliefs and behaviours.

Peer group pressure and its influence on health behaviour

As well as our personalities and our families influencing our attitudes to health as we grow up, and in adulthood, our peers are an important factor in helping to shape our beliefs. We share ideas with those around us, and most people feel a need to conform to the social groups to which they feel some attachment, and an important way of 'fitting in' is to share similar thoughts, beliefs and behaviour. Smoking is a good example. Although there is much evidence that smoking parents and siblings are associated with a two- to fourfold increased likelihood of smoking in children from the same household, outside the home the factor most strongly associated with the uptake of smoking is peer group pressure (Swan *et al.*, 1989). This review of the literature also noted that although girls were more aware of the health hazards of smoking than boys, girls were more likely to think that young smokers appeared more 'grown up'. Young girls may also believe that smoking helps weight control.

Peer pressure also plays its part in adulthood. Jones and Belsey (1977) looked at factors which they felt influenced the high breastfeeding rates in Lambeth, London, and felt that the example set by the large local immigrant population was a major factor. More recently Gregg (1989) looked at the attitudes of teenagers in Liverpool to breastfeeding, where the uptake rate is only 30-35 per cent and found that although three-quarters of the sample described breastfeeding as more natural and healthier for the baby, 36 per cent felt bottlefeeding was more 'modern', 15 per cent felt that seeing a woman breastfeed would remind them of topless sexual images of women, 11 per cent thought breasts were 'rude' and 8 per cent thought that breastfeeding was 'rude'. Although it is difficult to be entirely certain where such attitudes originate and how they become culturally widespread, it would seem reasonable to assume that the teenagers felt 'safe' in their answers as these were shared with their friends and possibly families.

The attempts of the midwife to encourage healthy behaviour will to some extent be offset by the social needs of women to conform to their social group. A change in belief or behaviour may be hampered by a more overwhelming need to be accepted by friends and peers. Peer pressure helps form beliefs in childhood, and it is to some extent responsible for attitudes and behaviour which continue in adulthood.

From a health promotional aspect, should the midwife attempt to change the attitudes and behaviour of a woman who is clearly conforming to her peer group in behaving in a certain way? To encourage behaviour which may reduce the woman's popularity, and therefore perhaps social support, may provoke severe stress. More likely, the woman will simply ignore the advice. The concept of peer group pressure is especially pertinent for midwives and other health professionals in considering matters such as sex education and teenage pregnancy, where friends and social contacts also influence behaviour in major ways. While presenting an ethical dilemma to the midwife, the task of challenging peer pressure may be more usefully addressed through community education and action, where change may be slow but where general attitudes which fuel peer pressure and the need for conformity can be addressed more fully.

Cultural influences on health

Culture is frequently mentioned as a major influence on the way in which health and illness are viewed and experienced. Yet culture is one of the hardest concepts to define in health care. To many of us the word 'culture' will conjure up ideas of ethnic or racial groupings but we often also talk of 'a medical culture' or 'a midwifery culture' and this suggests that every broad social or profession group with which we identify will influence our lives. This can occur in very sophisticated, subconscious ways.

Culture is seen by social anthropologists as the fabric of beliefs of a society, involving religious beliefs, myths, art, manners, dress, etc., which holds that society together and is transmitted through the generations in spoken and unspoken ways. The words 'society' and 'culture' run together. Culture is a part of society, but the same, or a similar culture can span more than one society. Members of a society tend to live together, or at least have close proximity to each other, while members of a culture share ideas and meanings which decide to some extent their beliefs and behaviour, but may be widely spread geographically. Society may therefore be perceived as more tangible than culture.

All societies have more than one culture within them; Helman (1994) states that most societies display social stratification such as class, caste or rank and each stratum has its own distinctive cultural attributes such as the use of language, dress style, and dietary and housing patterns. Helman also refers to subcultures and lists as examples the medical, nursing, legal and military professions, each with their own rules, language, behaviour and social organization. As well as sharing many values of the larger culture, the subculture forms its own distinctive boundaries.

The functions of cultures and subcultures are manifold. Perhaps one of the most important is the sense of belonging, which is gained from sharing beliefs, behaviours, knowledge, art and/or customs, etc. Humans are social animals and cultural ties strengthen the self-esteem of the cultural group, and that of the individuals within it.

Our culture also teaches us how to perceive and interpret the world around us, within the framework of the specific set of shared meanings. It also teaches us how to understand ourselves and justifies our conduct to ourselves.

Historically, belonging within a culture no doubt helped the evolutionary process in group survival and defence by the pursuit of common goals by a homogeneous group of people.

Subcultures often reinforce the social stratification in the larger culture and attempt to maintain a hierarchy by making differences between various subcultures explicit. For instance, the wearing of uniform or a distinguishing feature such as hanging a stethoscope around one's neck, sends messages to others about one's position or responsibility within that subculture or organization. Within a hospital subculture, encouraging inpatients to dress in nightwear during the day also sends strong messages about the holders of power and status, although very practical reasons for clothing and the way it is worn also exist.

There are dangers in health professionals being unaware of, or misunderstanding a culture, or its manifestation in behaviour. Perhaps the most serious is that of stereotyping people, when it is assumed that a culture makes all members of the cultural group think, feel and behave in a certain way. There are many individual factors, such as age, gender, personality and education which influence the way we make our decisions, as well as social factors such as class and economic status. Furthermore, a danger exists if the midwife or health professional puts individuals' health problems down to their culture and ignores an entirely different cause – such as a social or medical one. Examples may be a family group of recent immigrants living together in a small space which is judged to be unhealthy by a health professional who perceives that the overcrowding (in her view) occurs from cultural preference rather than economic necessity; or the issue of the cultural interpretation of pain, where the representatives of one culture feel that representatives of a different cultural group 'act out' pain, therefore making it less physically felt, and assuming a lower requirement for analgesia.

In the multi-ethnic Britain of today, health professionals would be unwise to assume that all people of a similar or racial background share a common culture. People of Asian or African descent, for instance, are made up of many different communities and two Asian women living next door to each other in Britain may be as different from each other as, for example, a Finnish and a Welsh woman in language, customs and beliefs, while appearing similar in looks and manner.

Immigrant communities change over time, and a culture is never static. Major changes can be seen with each generation, as children are educated in the country of their parents' adopted home. Indeed, if born in the new country these children are not immigrants. It does not necessarily take a generation for the outlook of an individual or cultural group to change, although change is usually subtle, and assimilation gradual.

Providing midwifery care for different cultural groups

When people from different cultures meet, first impressions and ideas are formed which will often persist in future encounters of the people concerned.

It is well documented that the geographical migration of people entering a country with an entirely different culture is stressful (Helman, 1990) and is often accompanied by an increase in mental and physical illness. Although leaving one's roots and loved ones is likely to be one of the reasons, moving to uncharted territory itself is stressful and one facet of this is living amidst an alien culture.

Helman also suggests that especially in urban areas, general practitioners may have among their patients foreign tourists and business people, students, migrant workers, au pairs, immigrants and refugees. Midwives too will be front-line points of contact, and possibly one of the earliest contacts for women and families with a different cultural outlook from their own. The quality of care provided will be partly dependent on the health professional's understanding of general issues of culture, as well as specific issues pertinent to that woman and her family.

The lack of a shared language is a major problem in the health care of women experiencing pregnancy and childbirth in a culture alien to their own. Although interpreters can sometimes be found, many consultations lack such an advantage and, anyway, having to repeat each sentence twice in effect reduces the amount of time for information-sharing by half, thereby reducing the depth of encounters with health professionals. MacVicar (1990), in a study of the health needs of Asians living in Leicestershire, found that the ability to converse in English was often related to the degree of integration within the community, and social isolation was more common where language could not be shared. In practical terms, what the midwife will observe is that the women who speak English usually lead more independent lives and work outside the home and therefore have better access to information and the health services. However even women with a good grasp of English may be flummoxed by the use of colloquialisms, jargon and 'hospital' language. Words such as 'fetus', 'antenatal' and 'contraction' which slip off midwives' tongues do not often occur in day-to-day conversation and may not be familiar to women with an otherwise very good grasp of the English language. For women with poor or no understanding of English, who are perhaps most in need of information and support, the barriers to a meaningful relationship with a midwife (unless the midwife speaks the woman's language, or an interpreter can be provided and extra time allocated to consultation) are almost insurmountable.

More specifically, problems related to cultural custom and beliefs may include religious or cultural rejection of fetal screening tests, any antenatal care, the preference for female attendants and the rejection of Western diet in hospital, or visiting times which restrict continual access to the extended family. Cultural needs can present deep problems in the provision of good health care and are as yet poorly addressed for all recipients of the health services.

Link workers are a relatively recent development in helping communication between the pregnant Asian woman and health workers (MacVicar, 1990). Their role is not only to act as an interpreter, but also to give guidance by education on such matters as the role of antenatal care, care of the baby and contraception.

In many cultures early arranged marriage and immediate pregnancy are encouraged. For the young bride with a new husband, extended family and perhaps new country, pregnancy and British health care must seem a frightening and perplexing environment rather than a supportive framework of care. In such cases midwifery skills are at their most stretched and challenged.

Midwives cannot hope to understand all the cultural aspects of all women's lives. However, by listening, observing, respecting other people's customs and beliefs, and keeping any questions open-ended, the provision of a service that meets the needs of all society's members is more likely to be achieved.

Early educational influences on health

Educating young people early about health can lead to future improvements in their well-being. Health education has been incorporated into the school curriculum since the 1970s, but where historically children received straight information on such aspects as hygiene and physical fitness, today there is more emphasis on promoting a more healthy lifestyle, with more focus on attitudes, values and skills (Cribb, 1986). Iverson (1992) has formulated a number of research-based principles which highlight, from the evidence of recent literature, the actions most successful in modifying health behaviour. He states that school health education programmes produce the greatest positive effects in children when they are based on skills training, peer involvement, selected components of social learning theory and involvement of the community. Using a number of studies to explain and support his principle, Iverson lists the approaches which have been shown to be effective in achieving behaviour changes among school-age children (modified in this list for clarity).

- Health education programmes designed to increase the student's basic life skills and personal competencies in coping with social influences – with interactive teaching and learning and student participation.
- Peer-led programmes focusing on social influences – for instance students talking about the feelings aroused by peer pressure, and the effect of the media and advertising on smoking, alcohol, etc.
- Programmes based on development of interpersonal skills – especially in groups, with students discussing for instance conformity and non-conformity, tolerance and personal differences.

- Programmes based on social pressure resistance skills – so students can feel confident about resisting behaviour they do not feel comfortable about, while investigating ways together of not losing their friends who may choose to behave differently.
- Programmes focusing on stress management skills, decision-making skills or goal-setting skills – so students can learn about the reality of making their own decisions and living with the consequences comfortably.
- Activities intended to increase levels of self-esteem – for instance students taking part in exercises designed to help them to understand their own self-image, practising role-play in giving positive feedback, and justifying their own decision-making in a supportive environment.
- In smoking prevention programmes, approaches dealing with peer pressure resistance training, correction of normative expectations, inoculation against mass media influences, information about parental and other adult influences, and peer leadership.

Undoubtedly school health education is becoming increasingly sophisticated and this will impact (if it has not done so already) on the way adolescents and adults respond to and influence how health promotional activities are delivered in the maternity and health services.

Summary of key points

- Personality has genetic, social and environmental elements and is crucial to the way health, ill-health, childbirth and parenthood are interpreted.
- Psychologists such as Sigmund Freud, Abraham Maslow and Carl Rogers have attempted to understand and form theories about personality development. A basic knowledge of such popular theories can help midwives to see where each woman is coming from and to individualize her health promotional activities accordingly.
- Peer groups are an important influence on health, and this influence continues throughout life.
- Culture, or the shared beliefs, manners and customs of a society have important functions in binding people together and showing them how to interpret the world around them. Cultures frequently have strong beliefs and customs influencing childbearing women and birth.
- Midwives cannot effectively promote or influence health without acknowledging the differences and problems faced by women from the great variety of cultural groups living in the UK. Particular problems occur where English is not spoken or is not the first tongue.

The employment and training of link workers have attempted to address some of these problems in health care.

- Attempts to promote health at community level can and should involve children. Social skills training, looking at peer influences with children, addressing social learning theories (including the influence of culture) and community involvement, all involving the active participation of the children, have been shown to be vital in making school health education effective. Relating these issues to subject areas such as smoking, relationships, sex and contraception all impact positively on the well-being of children as society's parents of the future.

References

Cribb, A. 1986: Politics and health in the school curriculum. In Rodmell, S. and Watt, A. (eds), *The politics of health education*. London: Routledge and Kegan Paul, 100–20.

Gregg, J.E.M. 1989: Attitudes of teenagers in Liverpool to breast-feeding. *British Medical Journal* 299, 147–8.

Gross, R.D. 1991: *Psychology: The science of mind and behaviour*. Sevenoaks, Kent: Hodder and Stoughton.

Helman, C. 1990: Cultural factors in health and illness. In McAvoy, B.R. and Donaldson, L.J. (eds), *Health care for Asians*. Oxford: Oxford University Press, 17–27.

Helman, C.G. 1994: *Culture, health and illness*. London: Butterworth and Co.

Iverson, D.C. 1992: Programme principles associated with successful health education and health promotion interventions. In Heller, T., Bailey, L. and Pattison, S. (eds), *Preventing cancers*. Milton Keynes, Open University Press, 171–83.

Jones, R.A.K. and Belsey, E.M. 1977: Breast feeding in an inner London borough – a study of cultural factors. *Social Science and Medicine* 11, 175–9.

MacVicar, J. 1990: Obstetrics. In MacAvoy, B.R. and Donaldson, L.J. (eds), *Health care for Asians*. Oxford: Oxford University Press, 172–89.

O'Campo, P., Faden, R. R., Gielen, A.C. and Wang, M.C. 1992: Prenatal factors associated with breastfeeding duration: recommendations for prenatal interventions. *Birth* 19(4), 195–201.

Sloper, K., McKean, L. and Baum, J. D. 1975: Factors influencing breastfeeding. *Archives of Diseases in Children* 50, 165–70.

Swan, A.V., Melia, R.J.W., Fitzsimons, B., Breeze, E. and Murray, M. 1989: Why do more boys than girls smoke cigarettes? *Health Education Journal* 48(2), 59–64.

Further reading

Brown, J.A.C. 1964: *Freud and the post-Freudians*. Harmondsworth: Penguin.

Kelleher, D and Hillier, S. 1996: *Researching cultural differences in health*. London: Routledge.

Kirschenbaum, H. and Henderson, V.L. (eds) 1989: *The Carl Rogers Reader*. London: Constable.

Messer, D and Meldrum, C. (eds) 1995: *Psychology for nurses and health professionals*. Hemel Hempstead: Prentice Hall.

Oliver, R.W. 1993: *Psychology and health care*. London: Baillière Tindall.

Raphael-Leff, J. 1990: *The psychological processes of childbearing*. London: Chapman and Hall.

Schott, J. and Henley, A. 1996: *Culture, religion and childbearing in a multiracial society: a handbook for health professionals*. Oxford: Butterworth Heinemann.

3

Social inequalities in health – what relevance for midwives?

Awareness and a basic understanding of inequalities in health and health care are necessary to all those involved in providing a health service because the distribution of health care still appears to be dependent to a great extent on socio-occupational status rather than need. The inequalities – present from birth right through until death, from the planning of health care through to its provision and evaluation – are one of the great challenges for health planners and workers since the discrepancies between classes have been known.

The study of inequalities in health and health care provision

The study of health and ill-health in a socio-economic context reveals disturbing statistics and an enormous quantity of unanswered questions in the health and social sciences literature. Although this was suspected before the publication of the Black Report in 1980 (DHSS, 1980), this report has provided a landmark in the acknowledgement of the inadequacy of health care provision, and has galvanized many researchers to explore why such inequality has come about, and what can be done to make the system more fair.

However, the study of health inequalities is beset by problems for a number of reasons. The terms 'social class', 'occupational class' and 'socio-economic status' are sometimes used interchangeably in the literature although there are differences in their interpretation. 'Social class' was a term coined around the time of Karl Marx, a nineteenth-century 'founding father' of sociology, who considered the nature of human society and was particularly interested in the conflicts that arose within it. These were fuelled, he believed, by the opposing interests of members of the higher social strata of society, who owned property and made money through it, and members of the lower strata, who did not own property and paid out to the property owners. Social class is seen in modern sociology as referring to a hierarchy of power and social advantage and, generally speaking, values about issues such as education, employment and health are often found to be shared within each social class grouping.

'Occupational class' is an indicator of social class used by the Registrar General (the head of the Office of National Statistics (ONS); formerly the Office of Population Censuses and Surveys (OPCS)) in formulating the statistics that come through that office. The listing of occupational class groupings used by the Registrar General is given in Table 3.1.

Where the ONS reports statistics relating to households, the occupation used is that of the 'head' of the household – taken as a husband if one is present, and if not, the woman. Although it is not difficult to see how such a system has come about historically, its appropriateness to present-day health care, and the stereotyping of 'a typical family' as one 'headed' by a male is becoming increasingly dated, and more ominously, covers up the fact that there is no real classification system for women, many of whom go through periods of economic inactivity and partial activity as they raise a family, regardless of whether a man contributes financially to the household. The officially recognized occupational and social status classifications which are said to be representative of women must therefore be viewed with extreme caution. Having said this, these are often the

Table 3.1 Occupational class: Registrar General's categories

1 (I)	Professional (e.g. accountant, doctor, lawyer)
2 (II)	Intermediate (e.g. manager, nurse, school teacher)
3N (IIIN)	Skilled non-manual (e.g. clerical worker, secretary, shop assistant)
3M (IIIM)	Skilled manual (e.g. bus driver, butcher, carpenter, coal face worker)
4 (IV)	Partly skilled manual (e.g. agricultural worker, bus conductor, postman)
5 (V)	Unskilled manual (e.g. cleaner, dock worker, labourer)

Note: these scales are used by General Household Surveys and referred to as socio-economic groups.

only national statistics available on which to base evidence and health care planning.

As well as occupational class for married women being traditionally and currently based on the husband's occupation, until a few years ago single women were classified by their father's occupation. Although new criteria are being developed which reflect society more accurately, stereotyping families in order to measure certain attributes will always have its problems. Households headed by single mothers now form a significant stratum of society but these households are not yet fully represented in social and economic statistics.

If occupation of 'head of household' must then be used at present as the best indicator we have for analysing social data, it must be acknowledged that it is one of many, often interrelated factors which contribute to socio-economic status. Occupation does not necessarily reflect the household's income (or expenditure for that matter) and values exhibited by individuals and families towards such issues as education, health and long-term life goals are surely as important to socio-economic status as are the occupation of 'the head of the household'.

'Socio-economic group' or 'socio-economic status', relating to social status and economic position, is a broader term in that it acknowledges that there is not necessarily a simple relationship between occupation and social class or status (for instance some manual labourers earn relatively high incomes compared to some people in social class 1 and 2). It also acknowledges that occupational earnings are not the only source of income – legacies, dividends, monetary gifts, the use of a company car and a host of other factors can also influence socio-economic status. However, statistical tables sometimes refer to socio-economic group, status or class in their title, but then measure by occupational class – a common mix of terms, and one which confuses the real definition of 'socio-economic'.

Because several sources of information have been used in this chapter, different terms will be used but it should be noted that care must be taken when considering figures and statistics that are not wholly comparable.

Studies which have followed the Black Report, such as *The health divide* (Whitehead, 1988) and data collected by OPCS/ONS have demonstrated that social inequalities persist in health and health care, and that little is changing, except in small pockets around the country where imaginative initiatives have been set up by creative and dynamic individuals and working groups. Political action is persistently called for by various groups; yet there has never been any clear agreement about what change is actually required – the balance has still to be found between policy, economics, political philosophy and basic social issues, such as housing and welfare benefits.

Although tackling social inequalities in order to improve health is more of a collective, political matter than one that can be solved by individuals, an awareness of the issues in health and the provision of health services and existing inequalities can help midwives to direct their care proportionally to the women who need it most, both on a day-to-day basis and in setting up maternity health care systems which address social issues and which reach all childbearing families. This idea of social justice in health care is imperative if such care is to maintain ethical integrity. By being aware of initiatives that have been set up by other midwives and health care personnel which have been shown to improve maternal and perinatal outcomes, these examples demonstrate what can be done, and can be used to develop midwifery care in the future. Some such initiatives will be described later in this chapter.

Health inequalities and women

There are some striking differences in the health and health care of women and men which continue to show up in the literature. For many years it has been noted that women live longer than men. It can also be observed that women are much more likely to be diagnosed as suffering from mental health disorders, particularly depression. It is unclear as to whether women are indeed more liable to mental health breakdown, or whether they are more liberally diagnosed because of society's messages that women are the weaker sex and perpetually under the influence of their labile hormones and, by inference, moods. 'Women's problems', such as pre-menstrual syndrome, menstrual variations and the menopause, are frequently labelled as 'in the mind' – although men with similar mood changes are often diagnosed as suffering from overwork or unemployment stress. Gender differences are not new in health studies although their interpretation has been subject to the cultural bias, often of a sexist nature, by the researcher.

Women are also more at risk than men from living in poverty (Bilton *et al.*, 1996) because of their work patterns, poorer rates of pay and the growth of one-parent families, most often headed and supported by the mother. Poverty places people at greater risk of ill-health through poor nutrition, substandard housing and the stress engendered in trying to make ends meet from one week to the next, and this is particularly true for pregnant women whose own health and that of their children suffer. Dallison and Lobstein in a report produced for NCH Action for Children in 1995 found that serious maternal nutrient deficiency and general ill-health, lower average birthweight and more low birthweight babies (i.e. below 2500 g), were prevalent in families dependent on Income Support.

However, as well as being treated differently from men, women's health and health care has also differed according to women's socio-economic status, or occupational class. Many health workers have noted

Table 3.2 Congenital abnormality rate per 1000 live and stillbirths by social class for England and Wales 1992

Social class (defined by father's occupation)	Central nervous system malformations (rate)	Heart malformations (rate)	Cleft palate (rate)
1	0.217	0.579	0.217
2	0.231	0.401	0.224
3 N	0.242	0.565	0.242
3 M	0.415	0.694	0.272
4	0.367	0.768	0.314
5	0.843	1.091	0.347

Based on data from OPCS (1995a).

wryly that the uptake of preconception care has been mainly by the occupational groups at the upper end of the spectrum, who are least in need (Thompson, 1984). Supposing the aim of preconception advice and behaviour to be, at its most simplistic, the preparation for the birth of a healthy, term infant, this is already predestined statistically by social class (*see* Table 3.2).

Although there are a few blips in the social class rates of congenital abnormality in Table 3.2, and they are only crudely calculated (for instance OPCS figures for live and stillbirths are calculated from births within marriage only, and the congenital abnormality figures are from all births), the trend is clear; social class (used interchangeably with occupational class by OPCS here) affects the statistical likelihood of having a handicapped baby. Why this should be is not absolutely clear, as genetics have a part to play in abnormalities such as cleft palate, but the trend does emphasize the very complicated role of socio-economic status when trying to unravel the mysteries of the causes of and predisposing factors to health, illness and disease.

The uptake of antenatal facilities by expectant women is also class-related. Women living in deprived areas often do not find routine antenatal surveillance and education relevant to their lives (Davies, 1993; Merchant, 1993). However, not only do women of lower socio-economic groups not avail themselves of the health services in the ways that their middle-class counterparts do, their treatment once in the system may be markedly different. Arnold in 1987 found that in one hospital antenatal clinic which she visited, some obstetric notes were marked with a gold star on the front cover. The midwife in charge explained, 'Women who have gold stars see their consultant at each visit. They are from Social Class 1 and 2.'

Women's health and access to health care may also be studied from an ethnicity perspective. However there is a danger in making the assumption that people from ethnic minorities or populations that are not indigenous are all disadvantaged. This is patently not the case. Nevertheless, there is good evidence that racial prejudice is still endemic in British society (Bilton *et al.*, 1996) and there is no reason to suppose that the health services are immune from such racism, therefore predisposing those using the maternity services to an administration that is not primarily based on their health needs. Although it is known that some diseases are more common in certain races, for instance sickle-cell anaemia and thalassaemia, the relationship between actual health status and ethnicity is unclear and, as yet, poorly researched across all occupational groups.

Perinatal mortality, low birthweight and social class

Perinatal mortality has long been seen as an accurate indicator of a nation's health, as well as the quality of its maternity services. The most significant determinants of death from stillbirth and in the first week of life result mainly from low birthweight and congenital abnormality. *The health divide* was a follow-on document from the Black Report, commissioned in 1986 by the Health Education Council (the forerunner of the Health Education Authority) to update the evidence on inequalities in health, and see what progress had been made following the recommendations made in the earlier report. Its main author, Margaret Whitehead, reported in 1988. She concluded that the health and social inequalities reported on by Black in the 1970s had persisted into the 1980s and that 'there seems to have been little progress on the basic problems underlying inequality in health, or on the specific recommendations of the [Black] report'. Some of those basic problems, according to Whitehead, included the continuing higher death and ill-health rates in the less favoured occupational and socio-economic groups from birth right through into old age. They also experienced higher rates of chronic sickness and their children tended to have lower birthweights, shorter stature and other indicators suggesting poorer health status. She also brought attention to the greater physical and mental ill-health of the unemployed, working-class women, Scots and those from the north of England, and the ethnic minorities.

The Black Report had looked at low birthweight and social class, but Whitehead made a most powerful statement in her conclusion stating that: 'Low birth weight is considered to be the single most important predictor of death in the first month of life' (p. 235). Low birthweight could be graphically demonstrated to be class-related in 1980 (*see* Fig. 3.1) and this trend is still seen to the present day although improvements can be shown, particularly in groups IV and V (*see* Fig. 3.1). The trend remains more closely related to poverty than to medical care, although progress in

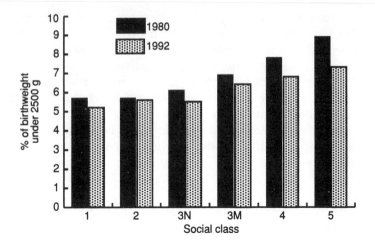

Figure 3.1 Incidence of low birthweight by social class for England and Wales 1980 and 1992 (Based on data from OPCS, 1981, 1995)

neonatal and intrapartum care, such as maternal corticosteroid admin-istration prior to an anticipated preterm birth to reduce the effects of respiratory distress syndrome, probably have a minor effect on perinatal mortality statistics (Crowley, 1995).

Cigarette smoking is known to be one of many factors which influence birthweight, and is strongly correlated with poor outcomes in pregnancy. Tobacco smoke contains about 4000 different types of toxic compounds, many of which can cross the placenta. Smoking can affect both the efficiency of the placenta in pregnancy, and the short- and long-term health of the baby. It has been conclusively shown to lead to intrauterine growth retardation and shortened gestation, both of which directly affect perinatal mortality and morbidity (Garcia *et al.*, 1994). Cigarette smoking can be shown to be class-related (*see* Table 3.3). Many health professionals

Table 3.3 Cigarette smoking status in women by socio-economic group in Great Britain, 1994

Socio-economic group	Percentage
1	12
2	20
3 N	23
3 M	29
4	32
5	34

OPCS General Household Survey (1996).

now argue that their time would be better spent helping women to give up the habit, rather than carrying out the battery of medical tests performed as part of antenatal care which are of unproven value, such as routine urine testing for glucose and protein by such unsophisticated means as dipsticks (where many false positive and false negative results are found), weighing women on a regular basis and routine ultra-sonography (Steer, 1993). This is a social issue as much as a medical one, and if midwives wish to address social inequalities in a practical way, encouraging smoking cessation is a good place to start, because it is now known that well-run programmes can be very effective (Garcia *et al.*, 1994; *also see* Chapter 12).

However it should be acknowledged here that even after life-style factors such as smoking, alcohol abuse and all other known risk factors had been taken into account and controlled for, Townsend and Davidson (1988:11) found that the health gradient between the social classes continued.

Explaining health inequalities

Despite the Black Report and subsequent studies, a number of questions need to be asked about whether health inequalities are real or a statistical artefact. Also we need to question, if they are real, whether people in the lower socio-economic classes are less healthy because they are socially deprived, or whether those in poor health move into a lower social class. Both of these theories may be true, and there may be further explanations of why social class appears so powerfully to predict health and access to health care.

Although there are a number of theories in existence which attempt to unravel the reasons behind health inequalities, a framework referred to in the Black Report (Townsend and Davidson, 1988) provides one such group of theories. While not claiming to be faultless it does nevertheless provide a background upon which to consider the Report's findings. Whitehead (1988) further develops the frameworks of artefact explanation, natural and social selection, materialist/structuralist explanation and a cultural/behavioural explanation.

The *artefact explanation* suggests that it is chance rather than fact that good health and social advantage correlate, as do ill-health and social disadvantage. Both Townsend and Davidson and Whitehead dispute this explanation, contending that there are now too many studies done from a number of different perspectives which demonstrate that however the figures are looked at, socially disadvantaged groups have poorer health than the socially privileged.

The theories of *natural and social selection*, unlike the artefact explanation, accept that health inequalities exist, in that unhealthy people move down the social scale, and healthier people up it. Indeed, there is greater sick leave in people in the lower social groups, and a correlation can be demonstrated between severe illness and hospital admission in schoolboys and their movement down the social gradient in adulthood from their social origin (i.e. father's occupation). However Jacobson *et al.* (1991) suggest that although social mobility is restricted in the less healthy, this is unlikely to make much difference to the observed class differences in health.

Whereas natural and social selection theories suggest that health can determine subsequent social position, *materialist or structuralist explanations* argue the opposite – that social position determines subsequent health, and particularly that poverty leads to ill-health. Much of this debate revolves around environmental issues. Whitehead refers to the conditions under which people live and work and the pressures on them, especially the lower qualified and least well-off, to consume unhealthy (cheaper) food, take on more dangerous jobs which may include exposure to noxious substances (such as asbestos or coal dust), accept lower rates of pay and live in poorer housing.

Cultural/behavioural explanations of social inequalities in health, like the materialist/structuralist explanation, agree that social position determines ill-health, but suggest that one's culture and/or behaviour results in ill-health, rather than the structure of the society itself. This theory argues that the more socially disadvantaged adopt more health-damaging behaviour, and have less concern for long-term welfare. In blaming individuals and their cultural background for irresponsible behaviour, the evidence put forward for such an explanation includes statistics that demonstrate, for instance, that more childhood accidents occur in socially disadvantaged homes than socially privileged ones, because the behaviour of less socially privileged parents is more reckless. It is also now known that widely distributed health education about the dangers of cigarette smoking has led to greater cessation rates among people from social classes 1 and 2 than those in classes 4 and 5. The reasons for this are not clear, but one possible explanation is that the culture of the socially deprived in some way militates against the changing of such a socially ingrained and addictive behaviour as smoking over one generation, whereas long-term health is more highly valued in the privileged classes, who are more flexible in adopting new values as the result of information and education which they believe to be correct. However, this explanation sounds much too simple and ignores the differences in access to education and affordable health-enhancing accoutrements (such as warm, low-rise housing, child safety equipment and fresh fruit and vegetables) between social groups.

Townsend and Davidson (1988) conclude that of the four approaches put forward in the Black Report, the materialist approach best explains health inequalities in their review of the evidence, but the other approaches may also apply at different stages in the life cycle. In the case of childhood accidents, for instance, the materialist explanation would blame the housing of poor families in high-rise accommodation blocks or run-down and poorly maintained housing estates with inadequate play facilities, more than the parent's social culture or behaviour. Whitehead, in disputing the artefact explanation, claims that there is substantial data to show that health inequalities between the social classes are real and proven. She believes that socio-economic circumstances play the major part in health differentials and individual lifestyle factors have little to offer in explaining inequalities. She also criticizes the artificial separation of materialist/structuralist from cultural/behavioural explanations, claiming these are heavily interrelated.

Both the Black Report and *The health divide* use the above explanations to attempt to elucidate why the inequalities in health and health care provision are present, and seem to be so difficult to eradicate. They offer a broad spectrum of interpretation of the results of studies into the health inequalities in society, and perhaps the greatest hope of understanding them better, and deciding how best to deal with them. However, this requires political will more than any other factor. Closing the gap of inequalities in health between the social classes must incorporate broad policies which encapsulate both structural improvements and policies focusing on individuals, and do away with the great class divisions so peculiar to British society.

The concept of social justice

It would be unrealistic to aim for every member of society to be in optimum health all of the time, but social justice should at the very least aim to ensure equal access to the health services for all, regardless of social class. However, this cannot be achieved purely by providing a level playing field. We now know that just providing services is not enough and that not all of the people who could benefit come forward to receive family planning services or antenatal care, however easy or open access appears to be. For some members of society, receiving free health care is secondary to more pressing issues in their lives, and in order for them to receive health care the service must actively seek them out. However, social justice then becomes embroiled in the problems of choice and coercion – what right has society to foist family planning or antenatal care on a woman who sees little relevance for it in her day-to-day life where her child's health, or her poverty and need to work long hours, despite poor pay, seem more germane? In practical terms, society seems to accept at the present time that it is acceptable for a health professional to go knocking at the door of an individual who does not turn up at the clinic to ensure that she is at least aware of her right to care, but there are only very few occasions where such contact should be taken further against that individual's wishes.

However, social justice in health care is about more than access. There is a need to acknowledge that justice means different things to different people, and in order for one person to receive justice, another may be compromised. Part of this debate now centres around health economics, in that resources are finite and cannot be stretched indefinitely. For instance, if a community midwife, during her working week, wishes to make four home visits to women who have not responded to invitations to attend the antenatal clinic, she will as a direct result of her extra travelling have less time to spend with other women who may have equal claim on her to explain tests, or perhaps discuss their birth plan. Seedhouse (1988) subdivides 'justice as fairness' into three types: 'to each according to his rights', 'to each according to what he deserves', and 'to each according to his need'. He believes that the third type, 'to each according to his need', is the most appropriate for health workers. Although in day-to-day work midwives must inevitably make subjective judgements about how they will aim to give social justice to all their clients, there remains a strong requirement to discuss the ethics of such decision-making with colleagues and clients, with the expressed aim of reducing unwitting (and deliberate) unfairness in delivering health care.

How can midwives improve the situation?

So what has gone wrong? The previous comments and statistics are a mere dip in an ocean of available evidence which demonstrates time and time again that access to, and use of the health services is dependent on social class rather than health need. Sir Douglas Black's Working Group concluded that the changes necessary to improve the nation's health were outside the scope of the NHS. People have other fundamental needs which they see as great, or even greater than health. These include social and economic factors such as income (which may be quite different from earnings), employment outside the home (or lack of it), the environment, education, housing and transport.

The recommendations of the Black Report included improvements in information given to the public, research and organization so that more effective forward planning can take place, redressing the balance of the health care system so that more emphasis is given to prevention, primary care and community health, and perhaps most important, radically improving the material conditions of life for poorer groups.

A number of maternity schemes have been set up since the Black Report which have deliberately tried to reach women most in need. The ones which have been most successful have had some similarities. For example, in some schemes

- the midwives, and often the obstetricians, have moved services out into the community so women have easier access to them;

- the women's social and economic needs are acknowledged and if possible met – they can talk about problems other than those which are pregnancy-related, and have easy access to social workers, housing advisers, etc., if required;
- the health professionals adopt an individualized approach to care while aware of and sensitive to the wide social arena in which people's lives unfold – with the woman being the central and most important character – not the hospital bureaucracy, or the health professionals; or
- attendance is linked with financial or material inducement – for instance cheap baby supplies, or free crêche facilities during appointments.

The Peckham Experiment

The Peckham Experiment was the brainchild of two doctors: George Scott Williamson and his wife Innes Pearce. It actually preceded the Black Report and was discontinued before the Report was even started, but is mentioned here because of its originality and success, and the important lessons to be learned from its existence. From the 1930s the doctors engineered a combined health clinic and fitness club which encouraged positive health by studying disease in the context of health, rather than studying health in the context of disease.

The health centre, built to reflect the philosophy of the doctors, incorporated a theatre, a gymnasium which included a swimming pool, billiards table and keep-fit classes, a children's nursery, a cafeteria serving healthy, attractive, basically priced food, a library and medical consultation rooms. At a cost of one shilling (5p) per week per family, all members had use of all the centre's facilities, which was open from early morning until late in the evening, and each individual had to agree to a periodic health assessment. Any people with serious health problems were referred to ordinary doctors or hospitals for treatment.

Doctors Williamson and Pearce believed that health in the family started before birth. Having worked previously with the socially deprived, they concluded that to encourage and achieve health in the poorer people in the inner city, preventative health care in its broadest sense, alongside medical care where this was necessary, was the answer. Ahead of its time, the Centre provided family planning and preconception advice. When a woman became pregnant, she was involved in a special consultation session to discuss the course of her pregnancy, diet and exercise, any problems arising from the conditions in which she lived and the place and conduct of her labour. Again, ahead of its time, her husband was encouraged to attend this and all further antenatal check-ups.

Consuming a healthy diet was seen to be a practical problem by the doctors for families which often lived in squalid and poverty-stricken conditions. To this end the Centre bought a farm in Kent where it kept cows to produce milk, and grew vegetables, which were then sold to the pregnant women attending the Centre at a non-profit making price. The Centre also employed a midwife who was responsible for advising families and providing antenatal, some labour and postnatal care, and the Centre doctors offered frequent health checks to all the children of the families.

Although the Centre closed in 1939 because of the war, it reopened in 1946 and ran until 1950. In its latter period of existence it added to its amenities a nursery school, a youth club, a marriage advisory service, a Citizen's Advice Bureau and a child guidance clinic.

Sadly, the Centre was closed shortly after the NHS came into being because it did not conform to the required organizational structure of NHS health clinics as it concerned itself exclusively with the study and cultivation of health, not with the treatment of disease. In many ways it became a victim of its own success – it was probably valued because the people who used it invested in it; one of the criticisms of the modern NHS is that too many people take it for granted and therefore abuse and overuse its services.

Writing in 1943 of what she learned from her patients, Dr Pearce said, 'Individuals from infants to old people, resent or fail to show any interest in anything initially presented to them through discipline, regulation or instruction, which is another aspect of authority. . . . We now proceed by merely providing an environment rich in instruments for action – that is, giving a chance to do things' (cited in Cook, 1987:126).

The Peckham Project was ahead of its time in its revolutionary ideas and practical philosophies. Its closure was a tragedy for the people of Peckham.

The Sighthill Health Centre

Sighthill was the first health centre to be built in Scotland in a suburb of Edinburgh, and opened in 1953 in an area of severe social deprivation. Its first antenatal clinic, separate from the GPs' general appointment times, commenced in 1955. In many ways Sighthill attempted to deliver a service similar to the model used in Peckham from within the newly born National Health Service. Its first annual report commented, 'The idea behind the health centre is to bring the different health services closer together, and enable them to co-operate to the advantage of the patient in the common aim of promoting health and preventing as well as curing disease' (cited in Dean, 1972).

The health centre provided GPs, physiotherapy and nursing services, child welfare and school medical services, dental services, a family planning clinic and a marriage guidance service from its early days. Antenatal care at the health centre was boosted when Dr Ken Boddy, a local obstetrician, developed a system of risk scoring pregnant women so that those considered 'at risk' could be targeted to receive closer scrutiny. The opening of the health centre in the community had already ensured that many more women were coming forward for antenatal care as travelling was much more convenient, often no more than a short walk, rather than a complicated bus ride to the nearest hospital maternity unit some miles away. The community midwives and GPs, when booking women in, would complete a 'schematic approach to prenatal care', in which characteristics of their present and previous health could be scored by numbers which would then be added up to calculate whether the woman was at high risk or low risk of complications, particularly perinatal death.

Risk scoring and targeting of health services at the time were thought to reduce perinatal mortality but this system has since been criticized for labelling pregnant women (all of whom carry potential risk from a medical perspective), and invoking unnecessary anxiety. It may be that perinatal mortality has been reduced so drastically in the Sighthill area because of the multidisciplinary approach to social problems as well as, or perhaps rather than, the medical approach.

The Newcastle Community Midwifery Care Project (CMC Project)

The Newcastle CMC Project was set up in the early 1980s as a direct response to the recommendations of the Short Report (Social Services Committee, 1980), which, like the Black Report but in less depth, had explored the relationship between perinatal mortality and socio-economic class, and found the results made dismal reading.

Two areas of gross deprivation in Newcastle were targeted: Newbeggin Hall and Cowgate. Newcastle Health Authority was particularly interested in the relationship between socio-economic disadvantage and poor pregnancy outcome, and agreed to fund four community midwifery posts so that the effects of the increased support which the midwives were employed to give could be evaluated by a sociologist. The project had two specified aims:

1. to provide enhanced support by midwives to childbearing women in their own home in an area of the city defined as having a concentration of high risk factors;
2. to measure the effects of this intervention on maternal, fetal and infant well-being, consumer satisfaction, and relationships between hospital and community services.

The project midwives were to provide a service which ran alongside that of the usual community midwifery service from the antenatal period onwards, giving extra support and care such as extra home visits in pregnancy and carefully designed parent education sessions reflecting local social needs as well as maternity advice. The midwives also worked closely with social workers and the Local Authority to help women address their pressing financial and housing needs.

Because the project areas were geographically defined, and because the midwives worked hard at making themselves approachable, they found that they were soon recognized and accepted by the local women, who became eager to approach them with information about themselves and their neighbours. Jean Davies, one of the midwives on the project team and main instigator of the study, described the networking as a fascinating social phenomenon which served an extremely useful social purpose in that midwives were given immediate access to knowledge about how women were, and where they had gone if they were not at home when a midwife came to call (Davies, 1991).

The project was evaluated in four ways: by case note survey to measure health outcome quantitatively; by client opinion survey which focused on women's opinions of the service and their health behaviour in pregnancy; by time budget study to look at how the project midwives worked and how this differed from the conventional community midwives; and staff survey to explore midwives' job satisfaction and colleagues' responses to the project.

The main findings of this small but significant study were that the midwifery intervention improved client satisfaction with the midwifery and hospital services, increased attendance at parentcraft classes, and encouraged reduced smoking and improved diet (Evans, 1991). Although the study was too small to demonstrate conclusively benefits in terms of perinatal mortality rates, it pointed to evidence of reduced incidence of low birthweight and reduced incidence of preterm delivery in project women. The data also suggested that project women required less pain relief in labour than control group women.

Evans (1991) concludes in her summing-up of the project evaluation that there are important implications for the midwifery profession. These include the ability of midwives working in such projects and delivering individual care to enhance the confidence and articulateness of socially deprived women in using the health services. She also highlights the need to ground midwifery in the communities where women live, rather than in hospitals, in order to be more aware of women's day-to-day practical lives and needs, and attract more women to come forward themselves for care and surveillance.

She recommends that midwifery education should include an understanding of social issues, counselling, group development work and theories of social policy and social structure aimed at enabling midwives to analyse the links between social issues and health outcomes.

Interestingly, when the initial four-year funding for the CMC Project ended, the Health Authority decided to discontinue the scheme. This decision met with stiff opposition from both the community workers and the women whom the scheme served. The women organized a petition and the project was reinstated, although in a much reduced form. This perhaps demonstrates that such schemes are difficult enough to set up; but continuing them, even when they are shown to be of value, is also a mighty challenge in the face of ever present political conflict and opposing interests.

The Albany Midwifery Practice (formerly the South East London Midwifery Group Practice (SELMGP))

Set up in 1994, the SELMGP was one of the first groups of independent midwives to be granted regional funding to provide caseload practice to local women. The team, originally consisting of five midwives, one practice manager and a women's health resource worker based in the socially deprived area of Deptford, aimed to provide total continuity by two midwives through pregnancy, labour and the postnatal period for 150 women (personel caseload of 35 women per midwife), thereby increasing women's satisfaction with the service and self-confidence. Now renamed the Albany Midwifery Practice and relocated to Peckham in 1997, the midwives have increased in number to seven and support 220 women at any one time. They manage their time by working 9 months continually on call, and then having 3 months off.

Because of their geographical location in an impoverished area of London the women supported by the midwives include a large proportion with social difficulties such as those from ethnic groups (including a Vietnamese population), women on Income Support, women with mental health difficulties, drug abusers and women with housing problems. The Practice liaises with a number of agencies involved with the women which it serves, for instance the Association of Women Refugees from Vietnam and mental health agencies. The midwives are able to offer free pregnancy tests, and antenatal care in the venue of each woman's choice. Following the antenatal booking the woman is encouraged to decide for herself whether she wishes to see the same pair of midwives, meet others with a view to changing, or pursue a conventional maternity care programme.

If she stays with the Albany Practice midwives, she will receive most if not all of her care from them (unless complications occur, but if they do she will retain her lead midwife) including informal, unstructured ante- and postnatal groups. The midwives aim to empower women in a number of ways. The group sessions, where both pregnant and newly delivered women attend, do not have a 'subject' at each meeting – rather, the women decide what they want to discuss. The midwife is there to respond to questions and provide information, if she can, when asked.

Women are encouraged to take part in decision-making throughout their pregnancy and in labour. For instance, the midwives are comfortable with a woman leaving the decision as to where to give birth, at home or in hospital, until they are actually in labour, and know how they feel to be in labour. The labour notes are completed to provide a running commentary of the birth process, often recording what a woman or her partner says, and how the midwife responds. As well as a communication record between health professionals and a legal document, the notes are a living, social record of what occurred. It is said that women are often intrigued to read and talk around this document after the birth; and many treasure the copy that they are given when the midwife's professional care ends. The second midwife at the birth will act as photographer at the birth if the woman wishes and this is practical, and a series of photographs of the actual birth, when available, can also give the mother a new angle on the birth, and a differing perspective of her experience.

Breastfeeding is encouraged during pregnancy, and postnatally support is given to each woman on an individual basis. The nature of this support, in giving the woman information and encouraging her to find out for herself optimal feeding positions with plenty of encouragement, leads to a breastfeeding rate of over 87% at 28 days postnatally, with a further 5% of mothers choosing to feed their baby by both breast and bottle (SELMGP, 1995).

The SELMGP is designed to empower a group of childbearing women living in a socially deprived area to take control in the childbearing experience at this important time in their lives. The hope and belief is that in helping them to gain the experience that personal control is possible in one area of their lives, they will be enabled to feel more confident and take control in other areas, such as becoming a positive force in their children's future health, and more confident perhaps in gaining employment outside the home when they wish. Further evaluation of the scheme is ongoing.

Summary of key points

- The distribution of health and health care in the UK is still dependent on socio-occupational status rather than need.
- Literature which assesses social inequalities in health uses a variety of terms, often interchangeably. These include social class, occupational class and socio-economic status. Care must therefore be taken in drawing conclusions from statistics which do not always measure similar data.
- Addressing the social inequalities in health requires an understanding of why they occur, and political action. Their persistence is partly explained by lack of agreement in and between the major political

parties about the severity, causes and effects of such inequalities, particularly for people living in poverty.

- Occupational class, used by the ONS to collect health-related statistics, refers to a man's occupation as 'head of household', or a woman's if she is single. There is no real classification system for women, many of whom go through periods of economic inactivity and partial activity as they raise a family, regardless of whether a man contributes financially to the household. This leads to particular problems in interpreting data about women's health, and no doubt conceals important information.
- There are striking differences in morbidity and mortality rates for women and men, and their causes of ill-health. Many of these are difficult to explain and where explanation has been sought, cultural and/or sexist bias on the part of the researcher or reviewer has often been apparent. The way society views women as the weaker sex, subject to swinging, unpredictable hormonal changes, may partly explain some of the anomalies between the sexes in the diagnosis of mental health breakdown.
- Women's socio-economic status can be proportionally related to health issues such as the uptake of preconception and antenatal care, birth-weight, and congenital abnormality and perinatal mortality rates.
- Although arguments have been put forward suggesting that health inequalities are statistical artefacts, reams of evidence have been produced to show that this is not the case. Some of the most detailed and convincing work is that published as *Inequalities in Health* (Townsend and Davidson, 1988; Whitehead, 1988, in a single volume)
- Midwives have an ethical duty to attempt to provide a service based on real health needs. To do this they must be aware of health inequalities and the way these affect people's lives. Access to maternity services should be under continual review to ensure that its services appeal to all sections of society, and everyone should receive fair treatment within it.
- There have been a number of projects over the last few decades which have sought to address some of the inequalities people face in terms of their health. Such initiatives, some of which have been described in this chapter, provide powerful evidence for midwives who wish to provide a socially responsive service, particularly for families suffering from the effects of poverty and disadvantage.

References

Arnold, M. 1987: The cycle of maternal deprivation. Abstract from *Midwives Information and Resource Service (MIDIRS)* of an unpublished article. Pack no. 4, April 1987.

Bilton, T., Bonnett, K., Jones, P., Skinner, D., Stanworth, M. and Webster, A. 1996: *Introductory sociology.* Basingstoke: Macmillan.

Cook, J. 1987: *Whose health is it anyway?* London: Hodder and Stoughton.

Crowley, P. 1995: Corticosteroids prior to preterm delivery. In Keirse, M.J.N.C., Renfrew, M.J., Neilson, J.P. and Crowther, C. (eds), *Pregnancy and childbirth module.* The Cochrane Pregnancy and Childbirth Database, The Cochrane Collaboration; Issue 2. Oxford: Update Software.

Dallison, J. and Lobstein, T. 1995: *Poor expectations.* London: NCH Action For Children.

Davies, J. 1991: The Newcastle Community Midwifery Project: the project in action. In Robinson, S. and Thomson, A. (eds), *Midwives, research and childbirth,* Vol. 2. London: Chapman and Hall, 104–14.

Davies, J. 1993: Mothers at risk. *Modern Midwife,* 3(4), 31–3.

Dean, R.M. 1972: Sighthill – the evolution of a health centre. *Journal of the Royal College of General Practitioners* 22(16), 161–8.

DHSS (Department of Health and Social Security) 1980: *Inequalities in health: report of a research working group* (chaired by Sir Douglas Black). London: HMSO.

Evans, F. 1991: The Newcastle Community Midwifery Project: the evaluation of the project. In Robinson, S. and Thomson, A. (eds), *Midwives, research and childbirth* Vol. 2. London: Chapman and Hall, 115–39.

Garcia, J., France-Dawson, M. and Macfarlane, A. 1994: *Improving infant health.* London: Health Education Authority.

Jacobson, B., Smith, A. and Whitehead, M. 1991: *The nation's health: a strategy for the 1990's.* London: Health Education Authority.

Merchant, V. 1993: Maternity services: antenatal care. The needs and experiences of some women living in two deprived areas of Lancaster. *Journal of Advances in Health and Nursing Care* 2(4), 79–93.

OPCS (Office of Population Censuses and Surveys) 1981: *OPCS Monitor,* DH3 81/4. London: HMSO.

OPCS 1996: *Living in Britain: results from the 1994 General Household Survey.* Series GHS 25. London: HMSO.

OPCS 1995a: *Congenital malformation statistics notifications.* Series MB3 no.8. London: HMSO.

OPCS 1995b: *Mortality statistics perinatal and infant: social and biological factors, England and Wales.* Series DH3 no. 36. London: HMSO.

Seedhouse, D. 1988: *Ethics: the heart of health care.* Chichester: John Wiley and Sons.

Social Services Committee 1980: *Perinatal and neonatal mortality report: follow-up* (Short Report). London: HMSO.

SELMGP (South East London Midwifery Group Practice) 1995: *Tomlinson substitution evaluation.* London: SELMGP.

Steer, P. 1993: Rituals in antenatal care – do we need them? *British Medical Journal* 307, 697–8.

Thompson, J. 1984: Pre-pregnancy care – essential for all? *Health Visitor,* 57, 64.

Townsend, P. and Davidson, N. 1988: The Black Report. In *Inequalities in health.* Harmondsworth: Penguin, 29–213.

Whitehead, M. 1988: The Health Divide. In *Inequalities in health.* Harmondsworth: Penguin, 215–356.

Further reading

Cox, C. 1991: *Sociology: An introduction for nurses, midwives and health visitors.* Oxford: Butterworth-Heinemann.

Dines, A. and Cribb, A. 1993: *Health promotion: concepts and practice.* Oxford: Blackwell Scientific.

Research Unit in Health and Behavioural Change, University of Edinburgh 1989: *Changing the public health.* Chichester: John Wiley and Sons.

4

Attitudes, values and behaviour

In studying and understanding attitude formation, health behaviour and the shaping of personal values, midwives will be able to deliver more meaningful health education and health promotion. Not only will a reflective midwife look to her own attitudes and values and consider how these affect her practice, but also the attitudes of women and families must be taken into account when providing effective care.

Why are attitudes and values important?

Everybody has attitudes. These reflect the way we think about everybody and everything in the world about us. Acquired as we grow up and develop, our attitudes are shaped by our family, our friends, our culture and our environment.

Our beliefs lie behind our attitudes. Equally complex, and shaped by similar experiences as attitudes, they are not necessarily accurate in terms of generally accepted knowledge. For instance, a pregnant woman who smokes may believe this is better for her on balance than not smoking because it may result in a small baby, and therefore an easier birth. This example brings us to the importance of values in understanding attitudes; the valuing of a small baby in this context, or an easier birth, will influence the attitude a woman has to, say, midwives generally, or the way she feels the midwives she meets treat her and advise her.

Attitudes then, are the result of the beliefs and values which we hold.

It is also important to acknowledge our own attitudes as midwives, particularly how we as midwives deal with people whose attitudes, beliefs and/or values are different from our own. Only by attempting to understand where other people are coming from, in terms of their beliefs and values (often vocally expressed as attitudes) can midwives hope to offer effective, person-centred education and support.

The relationship between attitudes and behaviour

Understanding attitudes has long been felt by many psychologists to be a necessary precursor to understanding and attempting to predict people's behaviour, especially in matters of health. It seems obvious that a person must want to give up smoking, or want to breastfeed, before she actually does it. However the reverse relationship between attitude and behaviour may be even more complicated. For instance, a woman may claim to value breastfeeding, and have a positive attitude towards it, without intending to breastfeed her own baby. The complexity of the issue is difficult to disentangle but theories to explain why individuals behave as they do will perhaps help us to design realistic health promotion programmes. Some health professionals still expect immediate behaviour change, for instance the cessation of smoking, when a woman discovers she is pregnant. It is known, however, from both observation and studies in psychology that for many women this may be completely unrealistic, as many factors influence such health behaviour. The clearer midwives are about these factors, the more influential they are likely to be as health educators.

Although an attitude is a *relatively* stable tendency to respond consistently to a situation (Roediger *et al.*, 1984), researchers have found over the years that attitudes by no means dependably predict behaviour. One of the most famous experiments performed to illustrate this lack of consistency in human attitudes and behaviour was carried out by La Pierre in America in 1934. He visited 200 restaurants and hotels across the country with a couple of Chinese extraction, with the intention of having dinner. On only one occasion did a restaurant refuse to serve them. When La Pierre subsequently sent letters to each establishment asking if they were prepared to serve members of the Chinese race, he received 128 replies. Ninety-two per cent of the sample answered no, and the rest answered that it would depend on the circumstances. Although the majority of the restaurateurs expressed prejudice against the Chinese and expressed their likely behaviour, their real behaviour when tested had been quite different.

Ajzen and Fishbein, in their 'theory of reasoned action' insert the word 'intention' between attitude and behaviour. They assert that by discovering a person's intention (rather than attitude), prediction of behaviour becomes more accurate (Ajzen, 1988). Figure 4.1 shows a modified diagrammatic representation of the theory of reasoned action for an intending breastfeeder and an intending bottlefeeder.

Ajzen and Fishbein (1980) have identified two of the many different beliefs that individuals hold, which they believe underlie any given action: those of behavioural beliefs, that is those which make us behave in a certain way; and normative, or desirable, culturally acceptable beliefs. They suggest that systematic psychological processes link these beliefs by way of our attitude to the behaviour, subjective norm (social pressure) and intention, each stage leading on from the preceding stage. Their examples are that people will reasonably take action when they believe the good outcomes outweigh the bad outcomes; and people will reasonably feel pressure not to act if they believe that people they are motivated to comply with think that they should not do so. In essence, people will weigh up their personal feelings, or attitudes, and the social pressure they perceive (subjective norm) in arriving at and carrying out their intention. Their behaviour then is one of 'reasoned action' (*see* Fig. 4.1). Although Ajzen and Fishbein suggest that their theory can be used to predict and understand attitudes and behaviour, the theory does not encompass emotional input, which is often unpredictable, and childbirth is not only a very emotional time for new parents, but very often an entirely new experience where fresh ideas and values are formulated.

Attitude formation

Although some writers suggest that attitudes are determined partly by biological inheritance (McConnell, 1980) it is generally agreed that attitudes develop primarily from learning, from birth onwards (Gagne, 1985). 'Learning' here is used in its broadest sense – absorbing what is going on around from talking, observing other people's behaviour and body language, reading books, magazines and newspapers and other general environmental influences, some mentioned in previous chapters such as peer and cultural influences.

Attitudes come about as a reaction between one's own personal characteristics and the social environment. Children are primarily exposed to the attitudes of their parents, close relatives and friends, and have a fairly homogeneous environment in terms of attitudes, values and beliefs. This is because when couples meet, each of the two is attracted to the company of another with whom values are shared, many of a socio-economic and educational nature, and so their children, whose early environment is closely controlled by their family and immediate friends, are exposed to a

Predictive behaviour of an intending breastfeeding mother

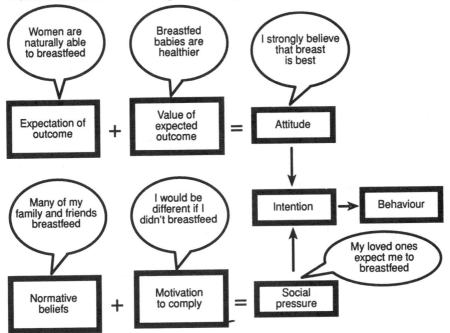

Predictive behaviour of an intending bottlefeeding mother:

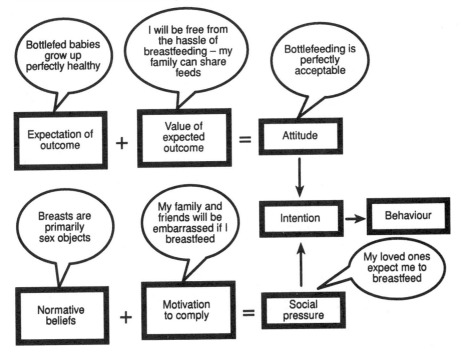

Figure 4.1 Modified theory of reasoned action (modified from Ajzen and Fishbein, 1980)

biased sample of life experience. The value of such early experience is in security and continuity at a time when the outside world would otherwise seem a place of mass contradiction and confusion. This selective exposure continues to be reflected in the attitudes and behaviour that the child expresses as it moves towards maturity. Sears (1969) has suggested that a critical period exists in human attitude formation between the ages of 12 and 30, during which time an individual's attitudes become long lasting, and after which they become harder to alter in a significant or radical way. Adolescence is a particularly important time for attitude formation, when strong social groups are formed.

Rapoport and Rapoport (1980) describe adolescence as a time of experimentation, excitement and turbulence, and a time for shaking off the authority of parents and teachers. They write of two phases of adolescence; an earlier subphase from about 13 to 16 years of age when young people push for greater independence from their parents but retain great internal conflicts about dependence and independence, and a later subphase, from 16 to 19 when they wish to forge a separate identity from parents and close family. These are essential stages of growing up, but in moving away from parental control adolescents will look elsewhere for confirmation of their acceptance within a social group. Usually the one nearest at hand is their peer group – similarly confused adolescents, also looking for excitement and approval, yet swimming in a sea of uncertainty about their personal identities. Normative and behavioural beliefs are aired and re-evaluated; sexuality and the new possibility of reproduction are often areas of great consideration and debate where attitudes are discussed, shared, formed and changed. Such attitudes and beliefs are not necessarily rational or consistent, but such is the nature of adolescence – the turbulence and experimentation require that young people try out different behaviours, different peer groups and different attitudes. Most will settle, a few years down the line, with attitudes not dissimilar to those of their parents, especially if they had a reasonably happy childhood.

Every social group develops norms and expectations which members are expected to adhere to. There is considerable social pressure for individuals to share values, attitudes and behaviours, and conformity helps to define the boundaries of a social group. People tend to mix in many social groups during the same period of their lives – for example family, neighbours, workmates, friends from school or a previous job, and they may be required to adopt different values for different groups. In order to accommodate these different values, people can live with a small amount of dissonance, or incongruousness (for instance a teenager may *normatively* agree with her friends that sexual freedom is a good thing, while *behaviourally* choosing to remain celibate for the time being herself) without feeling too uncomfortable. However, the need to conform to group order is very strong, and a discrepancy in beliefs and values between group members will often lead to break-up and reforming of new friendships where values are re-explored and shared. For the same reason, where friends or a social group have congruous values and attitudes, their relationship is likely to be long lasting, and add much to the psychological well-being of each participating member.

When a woman becomes pregnant for the first time, unless she is very socially isolated (a situation that may cause great psychological problems) she will enter a new social group of 'expectant mothers'. Many women are keen to look for information at this time about their new condition, but along with this information inevitably come other people's values and attitudes. Although the way women accept the new knowledge may be preset by their personality and social environment, major life events often bring with them the propensity for openness to absorb new information and new or reconsidered attitudes, in an attempt to become part of the new social group of mothers.

Challenging attitudes and changing behaviour through health education

Although it is important to acknowledge other people's attitudes and values in health education and promotion, and to respect them, it is also important that a supportive environment is created in which people can challenge ideas and question beliefs. The development of knowledge about ourselves and the outside world aroused by such challenges provides a day-to-day allure in life for the companionship of others both to confirm our beliefs, and when we feel secure enough, to move on to different levels of knowledge, with which come more complex beliefs and attitudes.

Expectant motherhood is a time of immense psychological development, when women acquire a great deal of new information, both from the experience of their own pregnancy and other sources such as family, friends, magazines and health professionals. Although midwives pay great lip service to the importance of giving unbiased information and respecting women's wishes, we also have a moral role in informing women about health-damaging behaviour where this may occur. Common examples include information about the dangers to the woman and fetus of continued smoking, alcohol consumption or drug-taking in pregnancy and making sure that women are aware and able to have the opportunity to discuss the advantages to both mother and baby of breastfeeding over bottle feeding. The areas of nutrition and exercise in pregnancy are less clear cut in terms of what is healthy, but nevertheless midwives have a duty to encourage discussion of such topics.

Education can be an effective technique in forming and modifying attitudes, and invoking more healthy behaviour. There have been a number of recent studies in the UK, looking at the role of parent education classes and individual tuition in increasing health by education. Hillier and Slade (1989) suggested from their study that women's confidence in labour and childcare was increased after attendance at antenatal classes, although the link between a confident mother and increased health behaviour is a commonsense assumption rather than proven fact. Knowledge levels in the sixty-seven women who completed questionnaires before the classes started and 8 weeks later, after they had finished, were also significantly greater, regardless of their occupational class. Although this study did not look directly at attitudes, the demonstrated increase in maternal confidence and knowledge gives weight to the argument in favour of providing education antenatally, not only to help participants to deal with the immediate challenges of new parenthood, but also to examine the areas of their lives where improvements in health behaviour can be pursued. In another study, Frances Evans in 1991 demonstrated significant improvements in health behaviour amongst women living on a deprived Newcastle estate when they were given individual midwifery support. Information was gained through a client opinion survey, where women were asked about their behaviour at an antenatal and a postnatal interview, by open-ended questions. In comparison to the control group, women who received increased midwifery support were better attendees at parent education classes, were significantly more likely to cut down on or stop cigarette smoking, and were more likely to modify their diet in pregnancy and the postnatal period in order to improve their health (*see* Chapter 3 for further details of this project).

However, the techniques used by midwives in educating women are as important as the information that is made available. The work and thoughts of Carl Rogers in the 1960s have been formative in understanding the importance of self-awareness and experiential learning in helping individuals to self-understanding and decision making (Rogers, 1983). This means that new information given to women should be tempered with encouraging her to express her own ideas, encouraging self-esteem, assertiveness and decision-making skills and using a wide variety of teaching and learning strategies to promote effective education and behaviour change. Indeed, in the Newcastle Midwifery Care Project, the informality of the parent education classes, and the focus on the particular needs of the women, were two explanations given for the high participation rates of traditionally poor attendees and their success in achieving more healthy behaviour (Evans, 1991).

In order to understand how people come to change their behaviour there is a need to differentiate between a change in attitude and a change in behaviour, and be aware of the time scale necessarily involved in moving from a belief such as 'I enjoy smoking and intend to continue' to

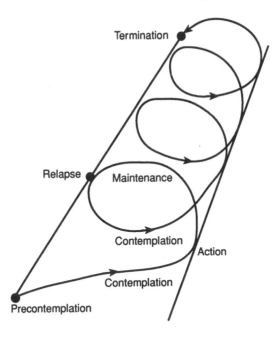

Figure 4.2 Prochaska's spiral model: 'progressing to the tower of change'. Cited in *Preventing cancers* by Heller *et al.*, OUP, 1992.

'I wish to stop smoking'. It is known that it tends to take an average of three to four attempts to stop smoking over 7–10 years for chronic smokers (Prochaska and Di Clemente, 1984). Prochaska (1992) has developed a useful model in identifying four stages in behaviour change: precontemplation, contemplation, action and maintenance. His spiral diagrammatic representation of these stages (Fig. 4.2) is based on his research that suggests that people learn from their relapses (e.g. of attempting to stop smoking) and each attempt to change behaviour takes them nearer to actual long-term cessation.

So how does this information help the midwife to lead women into making healthy choices in their pregnancies which can set them up for better long-term health beyond the duration of the relationship with the midwife?

Smoking is a good example of undesirable health behaviour that midwives often feel they would like to address with individual women in their care. To be effective, the midwife will need to find out first how the woman feels about the habit. Initiation of a discussion may lead to a number of responses in the woman. She may be hostile to any attempt to discuss the dangers of smoking, suggesting that she has yet to reach the precontemplative stage (and may indeed never do so). Realistically, it is unlikely that further attempts to discuss cessation will serve a useful purpose, and may even damage the midwife's relationship with the woman. Alternatively she may accept anti-smoking arguments but claim to feel quite powerless to stop. Here it will be useful to discuss the reasons for the feelings of powerlessness, and consider how they may be overcome. This woman is in the contemplative stage of cessation and may yet need to embark on a number of attempts before success is achieved. She may benefit from referral to a smoking cessation group if this appeals to her and fits in with her other commitments, but whether or not she attends she will benefit from midwives' positive encouragement and enhancement of her self-confidence in moving towards making a decision. Another woman may be at the action stage and have already cut down on her smoking, or stopped, but will nevertheless appreciate encouragement in her efforts. The woman who has made a number of attempts to stop smoking will have the advantage of learning about her limitations, but the disadvantage of previous lack of success. A pregnancy, or the thought of one, may be the motivation she needs to stop smoking permanently or for the duration of her pregnancy, although she will not know this until the baby is born. Finally, a word about the woman who appears to have successfully stopped smoking for some time: pregnancy can be a stressful time, and the temptation to return to smoking can be strong. Continued positive encouragement will still be helpful.

The Nottingham Mothers' Stop Smoking Project (Power *et al.*, 1989) combined encouragement, the use of a carbon monoxide monitor and the offer of attendance at self-help groups to pregnant smokers and obtained promising results in the evaluation of the scheme. Women reported very positive feelings about the project, particularly about being made to think, being encouraged to cut down on the number of cigarettes smoked and receiving good reinforcement in their efforts to stop or reduce their habit. Those who replied to a questionnaire 6 months after giving birth continued on the whole to value the support they had received in their pregnancy. The report noted that women who had managed to reduce or stop smoking in early pregnancy, before their antenatal booking, seemed to be particularly in need of continuing encouragement by their carers throughout the pregnancy to help avoid relapse, but because they often reported their early success at their booking visit, there was the danger that they were considered permanently reformed by the midwives and doctors. The Nottingham Project is one of very few of its type in the UK which has been researched and reported on, and it seems that an enormous challenge exists for midwives in moving into the area of helping pregnant women to stop or reduce cigarette smoking, now that evidence is available to show that planned programmes are an important part of antenatal care. They can be effective in helping women to reduce and stop smoking, and in turn may well be the most effective intervention we have to reduce perinatal morbidity and mortality.

Summary of key points

- Understanding attitude formation is a necessary prerequisite in understanding why people behave as they do in health matters.
- The relationship between a person's attitude and her behaviour is complex. In other words, expressed attitudes are poor predictors of future behaviour. This is probably because people's thought processes are complicated and receive such a variety of stimuli, such as new information, social and cultural pressures and fluctuating emotions, that consistency becomes impossible.
- Although attitudes may be determined partly by natural inheritance it is generally agreed that they form from birth, the strongest influences being family, peer and socio-cultural pressures.
- Attitudes fluctuate and change particularly rapidly in the teens when experimentation with many aspects of life is the norm for teenagers of all cultural backgrounds. However attitudes generally settle in young adults to reflect those of their family, particularly if their childhood was a happy one.
- First pregnancy is often a time when people are open to new ideas and may change their attitudes as they re-evaluate their lives, learn more about themselves and join a new social group of parents.
- The study of attitudes provides new information on which to take forward the move towards more effective health education and promotion. However because attitudes are not entirely stable, research on them is notoriously difficult to perform in a replicable way.
- Studies have demonstrated that effective parent education programmes which explore strategies to cope with new parenthood and offer emotional support can lead to behaviour change likely to lead in its turn to better health, in all socio-economic groups. It is also stated in the literature that encouraging people to express their own ideas, and developing assertiveness and decision-making skills are important in helping people to change their behaviour potentially to enhance their health. However, changes in attitude and changes in behaviour take time.
- Midwives need to be sensitive to individuals' values, the complex issues of health behaviour and the ethical dimensions of attempting to change other people's values and attitudes, often where optimal research evidence simply does not exist – and probably cannot, in the context of attitude studies being applicable to general populations, rather than to individuals.

References

Ajzen, I. 1988: *Attitudes, personality and behaviour.* Milton Keynes: Open University Press.

Ajzen, I. and Fishbein, M. (eds) 1980: *Understanding attitudes and predicting social behaviour.* Englewood Cliffs, New Jersey: Prentice Hall.

Evans, F. 1991: The Newcastle Community Midwifery Project: the evaluation of the project. In Robinson, S. and Thomson, A. (eds), *Midwives, research and childbirth* Vol. 2. London: Chapman and Hall, 115–39.

Gagne, R.M. 1985: *The conditions of learning and theory of instruction.* New York: Holt Saunders International Editions.

Hillier, C. and Slade, P. 1989: The impact of antenatal classes on knowledge, anxiety and confidence in primiparous women. *Journal of Reproductive and Infant Psychology* 7(1), 3–13.

McConnell, J.V. 1980: *Understanding human behaviour.* New York: Holt, Rinehart and Winston.

Power, L., Gillies, P.A., Madeley, R.J. and Abbott, M. 1989: Research in an antenatal clinic – the experience of the Nottingham Mothers' Stop Smoking Project. *Midwifery* 5, 106–12.

Prochaska, J.O. 1992: What causes people to change from unhealthy to health-enhancing behaviour? In Heller, T., Bailey, L. and Pattison, S. (eds), *Preventing cancers.* Buckingham: Open University Press, 147–53.

Prochaska, J.O., and Di Clemente, C.C. 1984: *The transtheoretical approach: crossing traditional boundaries of therapy.* Homewood, Illinois: Dow Jones/Irwin.

Rapoport, R. and Rapoport, R. 1980: *Growing through life.* London: Harper and Row.

Roediger, H.L., Rushton, J.P., Capaldi, E.D. and Paris, S.G. 1998: *Psychology.* Boston: Little and Brown.

Rogers, C.R. 1983: *Freedom to learn in the 1980's.* Ohio: Bell and Howell.

Sears, D.O. 1969: Political behaviour. In Lindzey, G. and Aronson, E. (eds), *Handbook of social psychology,* Vol. 5. Reading, MA: Addison-Wesley, 314–458.

Further reading

Combes, G. and Schonveld, A. 1992: *Life will never be the same again.* London: Health Education Authority.

Research Unit in Health and Behavioural Change, 1989: *Changing the public health.* Chichester: John Wiley and Sons.

Wilson-Barnett, J. 1993: Health promotion and nursing practice. In Dines, A. and Cribb, A. (eds), *Health promotion: concepts and practice.* Oxford: Blackwell Scientific, 195–204.

5

Using health promotion models and approaches in midwifery

Models have been used in disciplines such as science, health promotion and nursing for some time, but midwives have been generally resistant to their use, often claiming that the unique and individual situations of pregnancy and birth do not lend themselves to categorizing women and their needs, then applying a standard package of professional care. However if midwifery is viewed as a health promoting activity, then it may be that health promotion models and approaches can enhance the way that midwives deliver care by developing agreed research-based frameworks which, rather than labelling women, standardize good practice.

Defining terms

On perusing the literature from the various disciplines which use models, it soon becomes apparent that many terms of reference are used loosely and interchangeably. Examples of such terms are models, theories, conceptual frameworks, approaches and paradigms. A brief glossary of these terms in relation to health promotion is provided here to avoid confusion, although the terms 'model' and 'approach' will be adhered to in this chapter, unless an original author refers to his or her ideas by a different term.

A *model* is a single physical representation of a set of ideas, often diagrammatical, which provides assistance for our thinking and understanding of the underlying philosophical issues of both theory and practice. It attempts to be objective. Nursing has adopted the term very much (although not exclusively) to refer to the individualized practical care of patients, although in other disciplines, such as science and health promotion, it is used to refer equally to theory and/or philosophy.

A *theory* is a proposed explanation of a situation, which may or may not have been tested for its validity in relation to other theories put forward to explain the same situation. Different theories for the same situation may be equally valid, as the experience and 'truth' of one person may be different from that of another. Therefore a theory tends to be more subjective than a model, and a model may be said to be a concrete representation of a tested theory.

A *conceptual framework* can be a theoretical or mental structure, under which ideas are formulated. It is more primitive than a model, and stems from an individual's own early development of ideas, which may later develop into theories.

An *approach* literally implies a means of reaching a destination. Bunton and Macdonald (1992) note that it is a term in health promotion favoured by pragmatists, who focus on practicalities, and eclecticists, who mix ideas arbitrarily, selecting and combining philosophies from various sources. Most authors refer to a set of approaches that attempt to encapsulate different ways of reaching the same objective; in this case, delivering health promotion. An approach tends to be applicable to the philosophy as well as the practice of delivering care.

A *paradigm* is similar to a model in that it is also a physical representation of a set of ideas. However it can also be used to predict the course of further investigation (Bunton and Macdonald, 1992). It is an inherent part of a paradigm that the ideas are shown side by side, so that they can be compared and contrasted; hence the term paradigm map.

Why use models and approaches in health care?

All health care workers have their own ideas about how health care should be given, based on their own values and beliefs, and indeed no two individuals deliver care in exactly the same way. These ideas, values and beliefs develop with time and experience but it is important, when working in a team, that certain values are shared and made explicit, so that the carers can work towards the same goals, and the recipients of care can be clear about the standards and outcomes to expect. Good models and approaches are based on thorough, recent research and so the models and approaches not only standardize care, but also standardize research-based theory and practice. Much of the research conducted in health promotion topics has started to concentrate on changing people's behaviour, but morally health educators should only do this by well-researched means, hence models and approaches add to the moral practice of promoting health. Developing unified models and approaches in health promotion and midwifery can therefore help us to communicate with each other more effectively and strengthen initiatives which benefit everybody, but the more sophisticated ones also allow for individual expression in both carers and clients.

Applying health promotion models and approaches to midwifery care

Rawson (1992) writes that there are now over a hundred models and approaches to choose from in health promotion literature, and they are still being produced. This is perhaps testimony to the speed with which health promotion philosophy is advancing, and the need for theorists to develop their own framework to understand and explain, in as simple terms as possible, the relationship between the theory and the practice of health promotion. Some models and approaches are better known than others, often because they are more frequently quoted and used in the literature. The few described here are chosen because they are popular, relatively simple, can be easily applied to midwifery practice and serve to demonstrate how different from one another models and approaches can be, despite having the same general purpose.

Ewles and Simnett (1995) identify a framework of five approaches to health promotion.

1. *The medical approach*: The aim here is to prevent and rid people of medically defined disease and disability by providing 'experts' (i.e. health practitioners) who have made a study of health and disease and can directly treat illness. An element of paternalism (one person deciding what is best for another) is involved because patient compliance is necessary. Physical well-being tends to be the marker used to judge the success of the medical approach, with minimal or no reference to the psychological, social or economic aspects of disease cause and effect. There has been much debate in recent years on the role and place of the medical approach in normal childbirth, and generally speaking it is now being rejected by midwives and government (Department of Health, 1993) as a suitable approach for all women.

2. *The behaviour change approach*: Here the health promoter ultimately aims to change the attitudes and behaviour of the client. Again this is a rather paternalistic approach, as the health promoter sets the goals

but the end is seen to justify the means; for instance smokers are persuaded to stop smoking.

3. *The educational approach*: The true educationalist will give the facts and information, laden with as few of her personal values as possible. The recipient is trusted to use the information in whatever way she chooses – to continue with, or abandon attitudes and behaviours as she wishes. The educationalist's responsibility is to raise issues. School health education is said to be amenable to this approach. For instance, where sex education is given, pupils are unlikely to avoid experimentation with sex because a teacher tells them they ought to, but if they explore the issues for themselves and with each other, including the relevance of self-esteem and the influence of peer pressure, this will in all likelihood assist them in behaving in a manner with which they feel comfortable, rather than because they feel it is expected of them.

4. *The client-centred approach*: Here the clients themselves decide what the issues are, and set the agenda. They are seen as equals and the knowledge and skills they bring to any interaction are valued. The theme of self-empowerment is pivotal. Some aspects of antenatal care are amenable to this approach, in that although blood pressure readings and other physical observations will always be important and their interpretation will demand the expertise of the health practitioner, the midwife who allows the woman to lead the conversation during an appointment, or who starts the interaction with 'is there anything you particularly wish to discuss this week?' is moving towards a client-centred approach.

5. *The societal change approach*: This is Ewles and Simnett's only approach which does not directly concern the individual. Society is seen as central to health in that changes need to be made on social and environmental fronts, making health easier to achieve for the majority. Examples given are more no smoking areas and a reduction or cessation of tobacco advertising. Democratic movement towards such political action is said to make the whole environment more health-enhancing.

Ewles and Simnett's approaches offer a degree of impractical abstract theory, in that a truly educational approach, devoid of the health promoter's values, is probably impossible. However the delineation of the areas is clearly useful in developing health promotion theory, and helping health promoters to understand further their own personal outlook.

Downie and colleagues (1996), in their model of health promotion developed from earlier work by Tannahill, describe three areas: health education, prevention and health protection. The areas frequently overlap (as shown in Fig. 5.1), giving seven domains into which health promotion activities may fall. By *health education* they mean 'all influences that

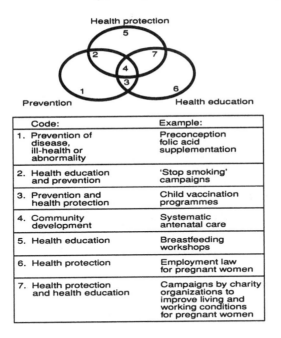

Figure 5.1 A model of health promotion (Reproduced from Downie *et al.*, 1996 with kind permission of Oxford University Press)

collectively determine knowledge, belief and behaviour related to the promotion, maintenance and restoration of health in individuals and communities' (Smith, 1979; cited in Downie *et al.*, 1996:27). This includes incidental as well as intentional education, and Downie and his co-writers also acknowledge the two-way communication process of education, where teaching and learning can come from and to both teacher and participants.

Health prevention encompasses avoiding, or reducing the risk of different forms of diseases, accidents and other forms of ill-health. It includes family planning, and breast and cervical cancer screening. Downie *et al.*, (1996:51) describe four aspects of prevention:

1. prevention of the onset or first manifestation of a disease process or some other first occurrence through risk reduction;
2. prevention of the progression of a disease process or other unwanted state through early detection;
3. prevention of avoidable complications of an irreversible, manifest disease, or some other unwanted state and
4. prevention of the recurrence of an illness or other unwanted phenomenon.

Health protection incorporates the environmental aspects safeguarding health by political, legislative and social control which use a number of mechanisms to achieve positive health by attempting to make the environment hazard-free, such as regulation, policy and voluntary codes of practice.

In their approaches Downie and colleagues include both individual and community action in health promotion but exclude curative medicine. They acknowledge overlap in all of the three areas of health promotion which they describe, and see community action as the ultimate in health promotion because it broadly incorporates health education, prevention of disease and health protection.

Ewles and Simnett's approach and that of Downie and his co-writers are two of the most popular quoted in health promotion literature, and others commonly quoted use similar ideas. The two detailed here differ in that Ewles and Simnett construct their design from the perspective of the health promoter, whilst Downie and co-workers' perspective is that of health promotion outcomes. Nevertheless, the two approaches offer similarities. Ewles and Simnett's societal change approach and the element of community development in Downie and colleagues' model have much in common in that they both encourage community-based health care with attention being paid to, for instance, the potential dangers of pesticides and of radioactivity from power stations, and the appropriate use of car seat belts and crash helmets for motor cyclists. Each includes an educational approach, although Downie and colleagues acknowledge as education all influences which lead to learning in clients and communities, whilst Ewles and Simnett restrict their definition of education to that which allows individuals to exercise self-development by deciding, without undue pressure from outside, what the issues are and how to interpret them.

There are wide differences as well as similarities in the two approaches. Downie *et al.*, do not include a medical approach in the curative sense (although they do acknowledge preventative medicine) and their model is distinct from that of Ewles and Simnett in this respect. The client-centred and behaviour-change approaches of Ewles and Simnett find no reflection in Downie and colleagues' model, who do not suggest how the outcomes of education, prevention and protection are reached. The major criticism of Ewles and Simnett's approach must be that in describing from the perspective of the health promoter, it does not attend to possible outcomes of health promotion, and the main criticism of Downie *et al.* must be that in attending to outcomes, or products of health promotion, the process by which success is measured is missing.

Taylor (1990) provides a more sociological approach to what she refers to as health education, although the breadth of her perspectives suggest that in today's terms she could be said to be referring to health promotion. Her ideas take the form of a paradigm map as shown in Fig. 5.2.

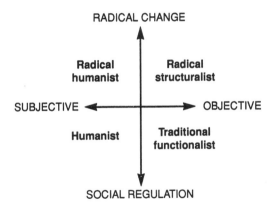

Figure 5.2 Perspectives of health education (Reproduced from Taylor, 1990 with kind permission of the Health Education Authority)

The perspective of *radical humanism* is that of self-development, particularly through personal growth but with outreaching effects for community development. Removal from social regulation as far as possible is necessary and in some cases health professionals may be seen as social regulators, in that they are required to work strictly to rules and laws. Self-help groups, such as the National Childbirth Trust and some support groups for parents of disabled children, are examples of the radical humanist approach.

Radical structuralism, like radical humanism, is about moving towards change in the organization of society, and indeed is more concerned with changing society to remove barriers to health than changing the individual. Examples include environmental initiatives to deal with pollution, and subsidizing healthier dietary options.

The *traditionalist functionalist* may be seen as the professional who possesses the expertise which is passed to the lay person, who can then progress to healthier behaviour. An example is traditional antenatal classes.

The *humanist* is concerned with personal autonomy and empowering individuals through life skills development. Examples are the use of the birthplan, or a health professional running assertiveness classes for expectant women.

We may look at Taylor's map in another way, by seeing how breast-feeding support can be fitted into each quarter. A group of breastfeeding mothers running their own support group could be considered an example of the radical humanist approach. Radical structuralism may be exemplified by a nationwide campaign to encourage breastfeeding, including legislation to improve maternity leave, an advertising campaign among the public to improve attitudes in favour of breastfeeding and the provision of widespread facilities for nursing mothers. An example of traditional functionalism is the existence of antenatal classes aimed at promoting breastfeeding, and a network of NHS breastfeeding counsellors illustrates the humanist quarter of the map.

Elements of other approaches can be seen in Taylor's ideas, for instance the traditional functionalist perspective reflects elements of Ewles and Simnett's medical and behaviour change approaches, and radical structuralism has some common ground with Downie and colleagues' health protection approach, in that it is concerned with political and societal changes to improve the public health. However, overall, the sociological background to Taylor's paradigm is so different from the more clinical frameworks set by Ewles and Simnett and Downie *et al.*, as to make these three systems impossible to compare.

Similar threads of ideas run through many of the published health promotion models and approaches but each has a different area of emphasis. Central to contemporary health promotion is whether action should primarily focus on educating individuals and small groups, or on restructuring society to benefit everybody's health, and this unresolved debate is reflected in the various models and approaches. The problem with focusing on individual responsibility in health is that the collective responsibility of health care providers can be lost, leading to 'victim blaming' or the scapegoating of sick or socially disadvantaged individuals, when health could be better improved for a greater number of people by addressing change in the wider society, by for example tackling and reducing poverty, or banning cigarette promotion in its many different forms. Therefore creators of models and approaches must aim as far as possible to design very broad frameworks which acknowledge the political dimension of health care administration, and also recognize the day-to-day practicalities for health promoters working with individuals in the community.

Using health promotion models and approaches in midwifery

Although examples of situations common to midwives have been chosen in this chapter in relation to a few models and approaches, it remains to demonstrate how overall midwives can use these approaches to understand individuals' different outlooks, and work towards a minimum standard of high-quality practice and common goals.

In looking at the application of health promotion approaches in midwifery, let us take as an example the midwives of Newplace Hospital, who note high cigarette smoking rates among pregnant women and wish to incorporate in their service a plan to reduce these rates, and to tackle the related problems of longer term ill-health and prematurity in the babies.

In formulating their action plan, they base their strategy on the approaches of Ewles and Simnett to take account of as many tactics as possible. Their interpretation of its application may be as follows.

The medical approach

Activities under this heading may include:

- offering smoking women examination of cardiac and respiratory function at various stages throughout pregnancy to check for and treat smoking-induced disease;
- advice to stop smoking;
- provision of neonatal intensive and special care facilities and
- collection and collation of national and local smoking statistics, against which Newplace Hospital can check its progress.

The behaviour change approach

Activities include setting up smoking cessation classes and inviting smokers to attend. Incentives for attendance and smoking cessation, such as financial inducement and free baby supplies, may be applied, the penalties for non-attendance or continued smoking being the withholding of such perks. The method used to achieve the stated aim of reducing smoking rates is that of persuasion, and facts and figures relating to the dangers of cigarette smoking are given to fortify women in their decision to try to stop smoking. (However, problems arise in assessing women's smoking habits. Should the women themselves be believed, when to admit continued smoking will deprive them of free gifts? Is the woman's peak flow monitor result to be believed, or her own account when these are in dispute?)

The educational approach

The midwives run into problems here because, in reality, they have set their aim to reduce smoking in childbearing women so they cannot exclude this personal value – that smoking is harmful and therefore bad – from their approach to smoking in pregnancy. A true educational approach is therefore not possible, because the women are being given value-laden facts and information, and not being supported in their own decision as to whether or not to continue, or cut down on their smoking habit.

However, while acknowledging this problem, the midwives could adapt Ewles and Simnett's approaches to suit their own ends better, and concentrate on 'an awareness approach' (rather than tackling smoking cessation) with women and their partners in classes or during antenatal appointments. Posters and leaflets about smoking may be displayed around the hospital. Women and couples could be encouraged to explore their own attitudes, values and reasons for smoking. Staff training and support will also be necessary, so staff are not drawn into coercing or judging women who choose to exercise their free will when this is in conflict with hospital's objective to reduce smoking levels. An awareness approach would be impossible to evaluate objectively because in asking women if their smoking habits were changing throughout pregnancy, this could be interpreted as undue influence (the women may interpret the question 'how many cigarettes a day do you smoke at present?', as, 'why are you still smoking, when we have made you aware of its dangers?'), and measuring an overall change in the smoking habits of the maternity population would not elicit which approaches had and had not been successful.

The client-centred approach

Again, the midwives will find themselves running into a moral minefield because they have already set the agenda and so the 'clients' are excluded from deciding what the issues are. A further adaptation of Ewles and Simnett's ideas is necessary if the midwives wish to involve people from the local community, which would be sensible. They may decide to call this a 'community involvement approach'. Activities may include contacting the Maternity Alliance, the local Maternity Services Liaison Committee, the Community Health Council and any other interested groups or individuals, particularly women smokers of reproductive age, who would be invited to comment on what initiatives they would like the hospital to institute in order to reduce the medical and social problems induced by smoking. However, asking such groups for their input after deciding to reduce maternal smoking in the area may well induce some heated argument about human rights (including fetal rights) and the role of the health services in prescribing 'good' behaviour to a population. A suggestion box in the hospital, for women to leave anonymous ideas, may get some interesting suggestions from individuals, but again this is not truly client centred; just giving token support to the idea of client involvement.

A truly client-centred approach could only occur if a midwife had no preconceived ideas about what smoking women should think and do when pregnancy is confirmed, and encouraged such women to voice their feelings about smoking. However when such a woman comes forward for antenatal care, and asks for help to reduce or stop her habit, the midwife can use strategies to empower the woman to find the motivation and means to fulfil her wishes. This may include giving the woman information about smoking cessation groups in the area. In this context, the client-centred approach is little different from the educational approach.

The societal change approach

Activities here are directed at the general hospital environment, and the midwives, in conjunction with other members of staff, are likely to designate all or most of it a no smoking area. However, decisions need to be made about how to deal with heavy, addicted smokers in the hospital who may smoke in unsuitable areas if driven to secrecy, and may dispose of butts in dangerous places. A smoking cessation course may be offered to members of staff, free of charge and possibly in hospital time, although this has implications for non-smoking staff who may see themselves as discriminated against. Problems may arise with members of staff who are happy smokers and do not wish to stop their habit, or more difficult still, do not agree with, or wish to take part in the hospital drive to reduce smoking among its users.

In considering such an activity as reducing smoking rates, it can be seen that planning the intervention using health promotion models and approaches adds many dimensions to the activity, and gives structure to its implementation. However, it also throws up many dilemmas, of a practical and ethical nature, that need to be resolved as the activity progresses (or better still, before it has started). Some of these problems take considerable time to resolve, and universal consensus as to how to go about the seemingly altruistic and admirable aim of reducing smoking rates and improving maternal and infant health may seem insurmountable. Without strong-minded and versatile leaders and players, this probably demonstrates as well as any argument why change is so difficult to implement in hospitals and health promotion programmes!

Summary of key points

- The application of health promotion models and approaches to some aspects of midwifery practice can offer a means by which agreed evidence-based frameworks standardize good practice.
- Terms such as model, theory, conceptual framework, approach and paradigm are sometimes used interchangeably in the health promotion literature.
- Models and approaches in health care can help us to communicate more effectively by concentrating discussion on shared values and beliefs relevant to professional practice, and putting these into a framework which explicitly states acceptable standards of practice, to both health professionals and the people in their care.

- Effective models and approaches serve to state the relationship between the theory and practice of health promotion. There is a moral requirement for health promoters (including midwives) to be clear about this relationship because where an attempt is made to change people's behaviour, as often happens, the ethical dimensions of such professional practice are immense.
- The study and application of various health promotion models and approaches to midwifery practice can help us to understand different outlooks and develop innovative strategies suited to particular communities.

References

Bunton, R. and Macdonald, G. (eds) 1992: *Health promotion. Disciplines and diversity.* London: Routledge.

Department of Health 1993: *Changing childbirth: Report of the Expert Maternity Group.* London: HMSO.

Downie, R.S., Tannahill, C. and Tannahill, A. 1996: *Health promotion, models and values.* Oxford: Oxford University Press.

Ewles, L. and Simnett, I. 1995: *Promoting health: a practical guide.* London: Scutari Press.

Rawson, D. 1992: The growth of health promotion theory and its rational reconstruction. In Bunton, R. and Macdonald, G. (eds), *Health promotion. Disciplines and diversity.* London: Routledge, 202–24.

Taylor, V. 1990: Health education – a theoretical mapping. *Health Education Journal* 49(1), 13–4.

Further reading

Tones, K. and Tilford, S. 1994: *Health education. Effectiveness, efficiency and equity.* London: Chapman and Hall.

6

Information technology and the media

Information technology or IT is appearing in almost every sphere of life and the arena of health promotion is no exception. IT is used to acquire, store, retrieve, process and transmit information both on people and subject areas. Although commonly understood to mean computers and their various parts, IT includes radio, television, video, and to some extent newspapers and journals. Of less professional interest to midwives, it includes telecommunications and micro-electronics, although we are reliant on these technologies in our work often at times without even realizing it.

This chapter will concentrate on the information technologies of particular significance to health promotion – those of computers, and 'the mechanical media' (Gill and Adams, 1992) which consist of radio, television, cinema, the press, etc., through which the public are sent a vast quantity of health messages. Both the advantages and the problems of the technologies will be discussed.

What is information technology?

IT is the mechanical and electronic means of communication. It has grown so much in recent years not only because of the great leap forward in the development of technology generally throughout society, but also because there exist a great hunger for information and a need to store and retrieve it efficiently. Books, videos, television and newspapers provide excellent everyday modes of mass communication but computers, telecommunications such as sophisticated telephone systems and facsimile allow us to make mass communication even more sophisticated, ever more efficient and sometimes more economical, although this benefit can take some years to realize.

One of the great ironies of IT is that although its purpose is to enhance the quantity of information communicated, it often limits the quality of human *'en face'* communication by substituting conversation for a machine. This point is of great relevance in midwifery where the quality of human relationships and communication is central to the essence of being a midwife, and a criterion by which good midwifery practice is judged.

The benefits of information technologies to midwives

Figure 6.1 illustrates the relationships between midwives, health promotion and relevant aspects of IT, particularly its usefulness under the various headings. The acquisition of information through technology has been a major area of development in recent years. There are a number of ways in which this is relevant in health promotion, both to the public and the health professionals. Perhaps the most common is through watching television, listening to the radio and reading various magazines, journals and newspapers. These are major sources of health messages for members of the public but although the mass media are good at raising awareness, they are unlikely alone to lead to long-term changes in the health behaviour of individuals (Ewles and Simnett, 1995). The value of the acquisition of such knowledge is therefore debatable. However, widespread public awareness of health issues makes people discuss them more and it is known that as a result some will, for instance, attempt to consume less cholesterol-rich food and lead more active lives, even for a short time. Therefore the acquisition of such knowledge through media messages may have a secondary effect in improving health – people do not respond immediately to the health education messages, but given time and the opportunity to redefine their own beliefs and change their behaviour, with the likelihood of further media messages and greater mass awareness, a few will do so.

Computers are particularly powerful instruments in gaining information, and are versatile in their usage. The acquisition may be by the public, or by health professionals who wish to gain information efficiently on specific individuals, or on general topic areas. Midwives often put individuals' health records at their antenatal booking interview straight onto the computer as the woman speaks, saving time by completing both tasks simultaneously. A further advantage is that the computer flags up

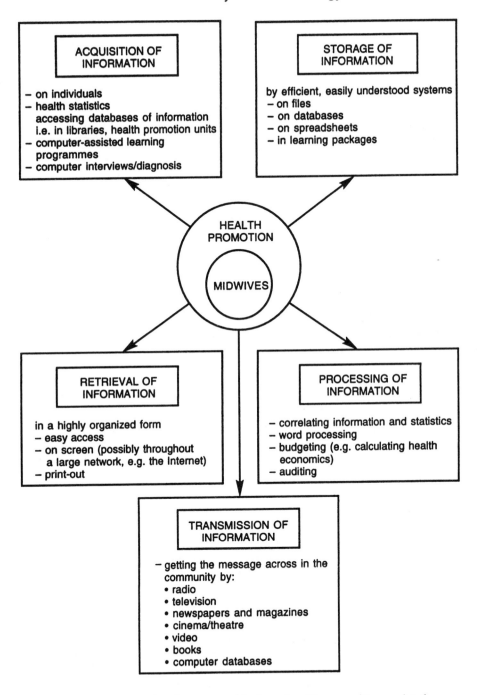

Figure 6.1 The relationship between midwives, health promotion and information technology

relevant questions, and can be programmed to follow up leads, e.g. suggesting a course of action if the woman smokes, or submitting a potential diagnosis if the woman describes a series of symptoms. However the problems of reduced eye-to-eye contact and the autonomy of the midwife in her response to the picture the woman presents to her are issues here in the critical analysis of such consultations.

Accessing databases, the organized information packages stored in the computer's memory, is a valuable way of acquiring information on general topics for health professionals and increasingly for members of the public who wish to increase their knowledge of health issues. Health statistics, for instance, are often available on computer where they can be neatly packaged and presented. The Cochrane Library incorporates a series of systematic overviews of studies, clinical trials, and health-related information formulated and stored on computer disk rather than in a book because of the continuous review of its contents, which are updated far more regularly than could be achieved with new editions of a book. The growth of computer-assisted learning programmes, where the participant follows directions on the screen to read about a subject of interest to her and tests herself on her knowledge (the computer providing questions, moving graphics and assessing the feasibility of the answer given) are gaining popularity, especially in nurse and midwifery education programmes and in schools. This growth may continue into adult education community programmes in the future, although the lure of television and its non-participant approach will always continue to be preferred by many.

Information technology is invaluable in storing the sheer quantity of health information available. Easy access depends upon efficient, easily understood systems, which the majority of people using the system can interpret. Here again computers provide a versatile strategy for storing statistics, learning packages, reference lists, research databases, questionnaires for general use (e.g. an antenatal booking interview), medical test results and a host of other frameworks of files, databases and spreadsheets, etc.

The processing of information refers to all aspects of the work possible on a computer but the processing of information specific to health promotion is worthy of mention here, because of the ways different aspects of health information can be correlated to provide new information, which would take many more hours to produce without technical help. For instance, if the relevant pregnancy and birth details on women are kept on computer, it can be programmed to correlate information on maternal smoking habit and birthweight, or other details, for both smokers and non-smokers. It may also be particularly useful in calculating local statistics for a single health authority or maternity unit, so that staff and funds can be targeted on needy local areas exposed by the results.

The transmission of information in the area of health promotion comes back mainly to the role of television, radio, newspapers, magazines, books and video, although to a lesser degree as we have seen, information is transmitted from computer databases. Getting the message across is done nowadays in increasingly sophisticated ways and even in television and other common media presentations, computers are used to provide sound or pictorial effects.

Getting health messages across via the media has grown enormously in the last 30 years. Media coverage of health-related issues occurs in a number of different forms, the commonest probably being news (for instance of a new piece of research), features or special reports, and advice columns. Many national newspapers and magazines have health pages, and almost every day on the television there is at least one health education programme. Even soap operas deal on a daily basis with contemporary health issues, for instance conferring on a member of the cast HIV infection, a newborn baby where infant feeding method becomes an issue, or a problem with alcohol. Although solutions are not necessarily offered, and 'bad' behaviours, such as smoking not necessarily condemned, these programmes are at least attempting to raise the issues so, as we have seen, playing a role in health education.

However, health promotion issues reported or enacted in the media are not necessarily accurate. Although it is increasingly common for health professionals to be approached to advise on the accuracy of information (and former health professionals to undertake jobs in the media), reliability and accuracy of information can be wanting, especially when the prime objective may be to shock and expose, or sell a product such as a magazine or programme made for television. This is an issue for midwives because newspapers, magazines and television programmes are a source of information for women, and in some cases for midwives, and if misinformation is given anxiety can be caused and knowledge and education undermined.

Midwives providing the health messages in the media

It is becoming increasingly common these days for midwives to be interviewed, or make their own comments on the radio, television or commercial video to communicate with large sections of the public about birth issues. This is a desirable development, raising the profile of both childbirth issues and that of midwives, especially if the presentation is done well and professionally.

There are a number of points worth remembering by individuals when appearing on television, radio or video.

1. Be prepared

Checking out the background

For people not used to being interviewed or giving a comment to the press, it is almost always a bad idea to give 'off the cuff' comments. When contributing personally it is worth considering, or checking beforehand such details as the name, subject matter and biases of the programme, the name (and if possible the style) of any interviewer, the likely audience so an assessment can be made as to the depth of information that would be most valuable, the funding behind the programme (it could be very embarrassing to find out later that it came from a tobacco or baby milk company, out to discredit health services), and who else is contributing.

Thinking about your contribution

Based on this background information a maximum of three or four points should be written down which are relevant to the contribution. Attempting to anticipate questions is also a useful exercise, and formulating succinct answers is the key to getting the main points across, and avoiding 'waffle', which makes listeners lose interest.

Writing the script

Health professionals are often asked to help with script writing of a commercial video on a health topic, such as infant feeding or the value of antenatal care. It is obviously important to have correct, up-to-date information on the subject, so pre-meeting reading is vital. Some basic, relevant statistics may be required although as a rule no more than one or two should be included as statistics are not memorable to most people, and can easily be mistakenly remembered (e.g. one in sixty babies are born with Mary's syndrome rather than one in six hundred).

'Writing the script' can also be a useful tactic when being interviewed, and politicians can often be seen to lead their interview, despite the perception that it is the interviewer who leads the way. However, proactively and doggedly sticking to one's own agenda for the interview requires determination, can look rude and requires a degree of confidence that most inexperienced interviewees simply do not possess. A list of main points, and practice presentations with friends, is usually a better preparation.

2. The appearance

Before going on air

It goes without saying that arriving early at the studio or set is important because late arrival not only puts everyone else's schedule out, but can leave the participant with no time to reread notes, use the toilet, meet the broadcast team and generally wind down from the journey with a drink and an informal chat with any other participants.

It is worth rechecking the earlier points with the interviewer or producer – the subject and length of the discussion, the main areas to be covered and who else is appearing. The Royal College of Midwives (1990) in their *Press pack* suggest that if the main areas of debate have radically changed since an agreement was made to appear, the midwife should seriously consider whether to go ahead with the broadcast. It is feasible to pull out of a radio or television interview even at this late stage.

The interview/broadcast

Appearing on television, radio or even in a professional video can be a frightening ordeal, even with the excitement of the challenge and the most careful preparation. In fact over-preparation can sometimes make it worse – knowing exactly what you want to say, but not being able to say it because of forgetfulness, or being asked the 'wrong' question by an interviewer can leave a participant speechless – the most terrifying situation for most of us! If an interviewer is present it is his/her role to prevent this happening by asking simple, straightforward questions (quite different from the role in interviewing politicians and policy-makers). If the midwife is doing her own presentation she is more likely to have a prepared script which can be read from, or the main points summarized on a prompt card or on paper to refer to if necessary.

The knack of a good appearance is summarizing the main points of the debate first, and embellishing them, if necessary and if given the opportunity, afterwards. The concentration of the audience is highest at the beginning of each statement or answer, and quickly diminishes the longer the answer is. However, the greater the wisdom, interest and ease of understanding of the first point made, the greater the likelihood that the audience will continue to listen, and gain more information about the point the midwife wishes to make. Also if the appearance is not live, cuts are likely to be made in the recording in the editing room, and short, succinct remarks are most likely to remain in the final edit.

It is important not to 'waffle' on a broadcast and when the point has been made it should not be laboured or repeated. If the recording is live the speaker will only be cut off, and if not, the excess information will be edited out. It is also important not to use jargon when speaking to the public because most people will not understand it and will 'switch off', probably for the rest of the programme. In such scenarios its use can be very damaging to health professionals, making them seem cut off from the needs of the public at large and functioning in their own world.

If, at the end of an interview the interviewer gives the midwife the opportunity to sum up her main points, the opportunity should be grasped.

After the interview/recording

If the midwife has made a live appearance on television or radio there is little she can do afterwards if she has made or agreed with a statement she immediately regrets. However, if it is not live, the producer or interviewer will usually offer to play the tape back, and ask for comments from participants, who may be given the opportunity to correct or rephrase any statements they are not happy with. It is quite acceptable for the midwife to ask that a recording be broadcast in its entirety or not at all, and that edits are not made that could change her fundamental meanings. However it is not considered appropriate that the broadcaster is asked to send the edited tape to the midwife for her comments once she has left the studio or set, or for her to re-edit what she does and does not want included. It is worth mentioning here that respectable broadcasters and journalists have nothing to gain from misinterpreting media health messages from health professionals, and tend to be universally helpful in guiding those inexperienced with the media, in maximizing their potential in the mechanical media.

Health dangers of information technology

There is no doubt that IT is here to stay, and will pervade all areas of our lives as time goes by. There are general dangers of the technology (particularly both computers and television) and specific ones, all of which require forethought in a quickly changing society. Without such forethought, and as the information revolution gathers pace, there could be social disorder leading to even greater problems because of the ways in which the technologies reduce human contact and divide society into the knowledge 'haves' and 'have nots'.

In increasing the time we spend with the technologies, we are decreasing our human interaction. Concern is already expressed in society with individuals, and particularly children, playing on their computers, or watching television, rather than playing with their friends. Technology often attracts people who find it hard to relate to other people anyway, and avoidance of human contact will lead to a greater number of socially misplaced individuals in the future, who cannot make long-term relationships or sometimes even short-term ones. An increase in mental health problems is the likely result.

The developing technology of the computer (it is predicted that in future, for instance, we will do most of our shopping and banking by computer) raises the following economic considerations which will have significant effects on health:

- Mass unemployment will increase as more and more jobs are automated. This is likely to particularly affect women, who are less drawn to computer work than men, and do more jobs at present concerned with office administration, much of which will be taken over by technology.

- Because of quick displacement of the workforce, mass retraining programmes will be necessary, and people may have to retrain for new jobs a number of times during their working lives.
- Decentralization of work will occur, with much more freelance work done in the home, leading to even less opportunity for human interaction, and increased social isolation. Gill and Adams (1992) suggest that the boundaries between work and home will become blurred as both will involve the computer. Therefore financial recompense will tend to be by amount of successful work produced, rather than hours worked. This will put pressure on people to work longer hours in order to achieve a better standard of living; they will have less time to socialize, and less time to spend with their family. They will also take fewer risks in the work that they produce, leading to monotony with working practices.
- Because there will be less work to go around, available work may start to be shared round. However this would require government legislation, as employers would tend to give all the work to the cheapest, basic quality tenderer for the contract if left to their own economic devices. If everyone worked no more than, say, a three day week (or perhaps alternated periods of employment with long periods of unemployment), productive leisure time would need to be reconsidered, and leisure facilities where people meet would need to be vastly improved. People would also have more time to devote to personal development through education.
- There will always remain a highly significant proportion of people around who cannot or will not relate to a computer. Although the young are generally becoming increasingly computer literate at school, some will always have difficulties mastering computer technology (as many do even now with reading and writing). However jobs will always exist for non-computer users, who will constitute socio-economic groups IV and V – for instance labourers and cleaners. Midwives, nurses and teachers, office workers and shop floor stewards will all be required to enter information on, and probably access material relevant to their job from a computer. There is a danger therefore that great divisions may open up in society between the computer experts, the key pushers and the computer illiterates. As the poor get poorer, they will not be able to afford domestic computer equipment and training (and many will not want it) and will remain unemployable except in the most mundane jobs. Without the implementation of a minimum wage for such individuals, the implications for the health and well-being of their families is vast, as we have seen in Chapter 3.

There are also specific physical health problems which arise from the use of computers. Long hours spent over the keyboard can lead to backache, caused by muscle strain, especially when desks and chairs are not of the correct height and distance from each other. The human body is not designed to spend long waking hours in the same position, and even with well-designed equipment, backache is very common. Frequent work on the keyboard may lead to repetitive strain injury, where the joints of the hands and wrists swell up and in the worst cases future keyboard work, or indeed any activities involving manual dexterity become too painful to achieve. Eyestrain is also a common complaint of people who spend long hours at computer screens.

Long-term exposure to low-level radiation occurs when people live and work with equipment such as computers and television. Although it can be argued that all electrical equipment, and even the soil (especially in Cornwall) emit levels of radiation, there are concerns about such artificial, continuous exposure. Perhaps we should be especially concerned for women and men who work with computers and delay childbearing until late in their reproductive life, when their bodies, and particularly their reproductive organs, have had many years of potential exposure. Meanwhile some trade unions and health and safety at work organizations are cautious enough to support women who ask to be given work that does not involve long hours in front of a visual display unit whilst they are pregnant.

Summary of key points

- Information technology is the mechanical and electronic means of communication. It includes computers, telecommunications, radio, television, cinema and the press. It concerns the processing of information, including its acquisition, storage, transmission and retrieval.
- One of the great ironies of IT is that although it exists to make communication of information more efficient, its growth and use lead increasingly to reduced *'en face'* communication by substituting conversation with a machine.
- Examples of the value of the computer in health promotion include its capacity for storing and correlating statistics, holding research databases and running computer-assisted learning programmes.
- The 'mechanical media' (for instance television, radio, magazines, newspapers) regularly raise and provide information on health topics. However, when the purpose of a programme or article is to shock, expose, or sell a product, the impartiality of the report may be lacking, and the public misled. Although the mechanical mass media are on the whole good at raising awareness of health issues, it is known that such

exposure alone is unlikely to lead to long-term behaviour changes in many individuals.

- Midwives have a role in providing health messages about childbirth issues through the media. However, in doing so they need to prepare themselves for the venture by both understanding the role of the media, and how they can most effectively use the time or space allocated for their contribution.
- IT threatens some danger to public health both physically and psychologically. Long hours spent sitting in front of a keyboard and/or visual display unit can lead to backache, repetitive strain injury and eye-strain. As well as leading to a reduction in the time spent in human interaction, which is likely to lead to an increase in mental health problems, the development of computer and telecommunication technologies will reduce the size of the workforce. As more and more work is performed by machines, the problems of increased unemployment will rise. The significant proportion of people who cannot or will not relate to a computer will be disadvantaged in their choice of white collar work, and divisions in society will widen into the computer experts, the key pushers and the computer illiterates.
- Midwives must be pro-active in keeping abreast of IT relevant to their profession and exploit the technologies for their benefits, while being also aware of their negative impact on health.

References

Ewles, L. and Simnett, I. 1995: *Promoting health: a practical guide.* London: Scutari Press.

Gill, D. and Adams, B. 1992: *ABC of communication studies.* Walton-on-Thames: Thomas Nelson and Sons.

Royal College of Midwives 1990: *Press pack.* London: Royal College of Midwives.

Further reading

Research Unit in Health and Behavioural Change, University of Edinburgh 1989: *Changing the public health.* Chichester: John Wiley and Sons.

Williams, R. 1992: *Television technology and cultural reform.* London: Routledge.

7

Evaluating health promotion activities

This section of the book would not be complete without a consideration of the ways in which a midwife evaluates how successful she has been in her health promoting activities. Whether she helps one woman to breastfeed, leads one antenatal class or sits on a committee which oversees midwifery activities at a local or national level, an assessment of effectiveness is vital in order to develop and improve herself, and provide an increasingly better service.

What is evaluation, and why do it?

Evaluation of health promoting activities usually involves two processes. First the activity is observed, and in some way measured. Such a measurement (and indeed the observation) may take on a number of different forms, but it is most easily achieved if well thought out aims and objectives have been laid down early in the planning process for the activity, with adequate consideration given to making these aims and objectives measurable. In this context, an aim may be defined as the ultimate purpose of the activity, and objectives (of which there are usually more than one), the way or ways in which that aim is to be achieved (*see* Table 7.1). Secondly, the measurement arrived at may be compared against an acceptable standard, or an indicator of good performance. A

Table 7.1 An example of a health promotion aim with the related objectives

Subject: Encouraging the correct use of car seats for newborns

Aim: That all newborn babies, when travelling in motorized vehicles, are correctly transported in a suitable car seat

Objectives: All pregnant women are shown a video, either in the antenatal clinic or at parent education classes, which demonstrates the importance, suitability and correct fitting of infants' car seats

All baby car seats sold must contain clear, easy to understand fitting instructions in pictures as well as words

An information officer is available at all times to demonstrate the correct fitting of the seat chosen by the parents for transporting their infant

Legislation is passed to make it illegal to transport a baby in a motorized vehicle without a British Safety Standard passed baby car seat

Police/court records are kept of the reasons drivers give for failing adequately to harness their infant passengers, and statistics formulated which can be used to evaluate the success of previous educational material, and help plan continuing education programmes for parents and guardians

quantitative evaluation, which usually measures the product or outcome statistically, lends itself to comparison with an independent standard. Although many 'evaluations' stop at the first stage, perhaps asking people how they feel about a health promotion activity, this is really more of a monitoring exercise which involves simply checking what is being done. However many health promoters involved in monitoring their own teaching and activities will have their own criteria on which to judge their success, and may call this process evaluation.

Evaluation may be qualitative or quantitative. Hawe *et al.* (1990) suggest that qualitative data are comprised of the range of and variation between responses, but that they do not record the frequency of response. Qualitative information, as the name suggests, is usually gained from the process of the activity – its quality in terms of reference to peoples' attitudes, feelings and many of the seeming 'unmeasurables' or non-comparable aspects of evaluation. Hence qualitative evaluation is often descriptive, the responses of participants valued on their own merit. Statistical tests are not always appropriate for application to qualitative data.

Quantitative evaluation, on the other hand, deals with the frequency of response – facts and figures are produced, which tend to measure the end product of the activity. The sample size is large and results are amenable to statistical analysis, for instance producing percentages or standard deviations (a frequency distribution demonstrating the dispersion of the figures).

There are many reasons why midwives should evaluate what they offer in terms of promoting the health of women, babies and society at large. Most obviously, it is because their activities may be useless, and a waste of valuable resources. At worst, their activity may make a bad situation worse. For instance a well-meaning midwife who, full of enthusiasm, launches into a discussion with a group of socially deprived women on the benefits of prime cuts of meat and fresh fruit and vegetables in pregnancy, may alienate the women and make it difficult for them ever to take midwives seriously again. Past evaluation and research has shown that health promotion should start from where the woman is, and not where the midwife wants her to be. Early observation of her interaction should soon enable the above midwife to formulate careful goals which reflect the needs of the recipients, and offer realistic outcomes.

Evaluation also provides the best sort of feedback on which to develop health promotion activities and methods. If the responses of recipients are considered as essential to achieving aims, their opinions and comments can only serve to help the midwife to develop her health promotional work, and the general learning environment she engenders.

Cost always comes into the effectiveness and efficiency equation nowadays and although cost should not dictate health promotional activities, it must have some bearing on whether approaches to improving and maintaining health should continue or not. Not only are resources finite, but allocation of funding to one area will inevitably leave another feeling deprived. The results of evaluation can help in deciding where money can best be spent in order to achieve the best overall outcome. Information on cost effectiveness will also be of value to service providers and funding authorities, in that they are able to use the evidence to spend more efficiently on proven effective programmes. An example of this is demonstrated in Chapter 12 where Val Thomas investigates how midwives can best help pregnant smokers. The Health Education Authority (1994) have taken account of past evaluations of smoking cessation programmes in order to put together an effective training pack for midwives and health professionals to achieve the highest possible success rate in reducing smoking rates, while being aware that midwives' time is limited, and could easily be wasted if midwives do not possess the information to help them gauge the amount of time they spend with each woman, depending on whether she is at a pre-contemplative, or contemplative stage of quitting.

Hawe *et al.* (1990) suggest as a broader aim of evaluation the extension of the literature on the subject, so developing further the theory of health promotion. This also ensures that theory develops from practice, rather than practice being decided by abstract, untested and unrealistic theory.

By having access to published data health promoters can be saved from reinventing the wheel. In setting up their own programmes, they can benefit from other peoples' successes and failures by doing a literature search and following the best evaluated practices and models, and also using tested evaluation methods which will not only give them good data about their own activity, but make it comparable, in terms of results, to the studies on which they have based their activity and evaluation.

Downie *et al.* (1996) comment on the need to evaluate whether health promotional activities are ethically justified. Aims and objectives almost always include an element of behaviour change, which may cause personal discomfort and have an effect on the recipients' relationships with family and friends. The effect of education cannot be predicted, and as seen in the film *Educating Rita*, where Rita's new knowledge leaves her abandoned by her husband and old friends and feeling misunderstood by her family, it can be a double-edged sword.

But once we have evaluated, why do we need to keep on evaluating? It is not enough these days to evaluate an aspect of health promotion, act to make the improvements required and then sit back and repeat the activity unchanged indefinitely. Health promotion as a discrete field of expertise is relatively new, and therefore its knowledge base is changing rapidly. Continuous evaluation and its concomitant replanning, and reassessment of recipient needs, will help it to remain alive, and adapt to the changing health needs of all members of society.

Challenges in evaluating health promotion

As yet, very little is known of the effectiveness of midwives in their role as health promoters. If it was decided that, for instance, financial savings could be made in the health service by disbanding Britain's community midwifery service, concrete evidence to support the continuation of the service would be hard to come by. After all, most other European countries manage without such an elaborate and expensive system, with little difference to their perinatal or maternal mortality rates (although many of them have more general practitioners per head of population). This is not to say that pockets of evidence do not exist that in some cases community midwives make a real difference to the satisfaction rates of new mothers, and have small effects on morbidity and mortality rates, or even that they do not make a real difference to health – it is just that most midwives would have difficulty proving it with convincing evidence and statistics. So some of the biggest problems facing midwives generally in evaluating their effectiveness are those of the size of the operation. Even for one midwife wishing to evaluate a health advice stand she sets up in a shopping centre, the size of the operation, in relation to the time available to her, may seem enormous. This is perhaps one of the commonest reasons for lack of evaluation, and tried and subjectively tested practices continuing with little consideration for their effectiveness.

Another common reason is lack of knowledge or confidence about how to monitor and evaluate – although even a short questionnaire can be useful in eliciting views and ideas of the recipients. Activities such as evaluation are often generally grouped together under the umbrella of 'research', a word which can instil fear and trepidation in people who perceive such practices as complicated and academic.

For a midwife measuring her own effectiveness in delivering a small-scale health promoting activity, reliability and validity are of little consequence. However, for larger project evaluation, these concepts must be addressed to make sure that results obtained are not spurious. Reliability, in this context, refers to the repeatability of the test. For instance, if a midwife tests attitudes to breastfeeding in a group of teenagers on Monday, she should get roughly the same answers the following Monday (providing there has been no intervening experience to change those attitudes *en masse*). Validity refers to the evaluation technique measuring what it was meant to measure. An example here would be asking individuals about the nature of their sex lives by postal questionnaire – the validity of some responses, especially where extraordinary feats of marathon sexual acts are described, suggest that ego is being measured rather than reality. Achieving reliability and validity can be challenging, and can best be done by choosing more than one technique or method by which to evaluate to see whether each method gives similar results. However, resources may not be available for small-scale evaluation to do this, and simpler monitoring must be resorted to.

There are also broader challenges in evaluation common to all areas of health promotion. It is difficult to separate out specific effects of a health promotion programme, and effects of outside influences. For instance, it may be difficult to discover whether women who cut down on alcohol consumption in pregnancy do so because of advice from professionals or because of what they read or hear from friends. Many women may not remember themselves with the passage of time and evaluation of the effectiveness of the midwife's input therefore becomes almost impossible.

It is also difficult to know exactly what to evaluate, and how. This will depend to a large extent on the knowledge and confidence of the health promoter, her resources, time available and support and interest of managers and colleagues. There are a number of ways of evaluating health promotional activities, and some of these methods are discussed here.

The levels and technique of evaluation

Once the broad range of resources are known to the health promoter, she will need to make decisions about what technique she will use. The huge range of evaluation methods referred to in the literature reflect the variety of activities, which all require some form of measurement.

DeBella *et al.* (1986) suggest a number of levels of evaluation, which are adapted and applied to some techniques of evaluating health promotion activities in Table 7.2.

Table 7.2 Techniques of evaluation and their use

	Interview	Questionnaire	Survey	Rating scale	Focus group	Diary	Performance indicators	Cost benefit ratio
Input Examples								
Facilities adequate?	✓	✓	✓	✓	✓	✓	✓	✗
Details of personnel, e.g. qualifications, experience	✓	✓	✓	✗	✗	✓	✗	✗
Details of recipients, e.g. age, social class	✓	✓	✓	✗	✓	✓	✗	✗
Process Examples:								
Teaching style(s) used	✓	✓	✓	✓	✓	✓	✗	✗
Content	✓	✓	✓	✓	✓	✓	✗	✗
Response of recipients	✓	✓	✓	✓	✓	✓	✗	✗
Output Examples:								
Number of recipients	✗	✗	✓	✗	✗	✗	✓	✗
Number of contacts with health professionals	✗	✗	✓	✗	✗	✗	✓	✗
Cost effectiveness	✗	✗	✓	✗	✗	✗	✓	✓
Impact/outcome Examples:								
Change in knowledge	✓	✓	✓	✓	✓	✓	✓	✗
Change in attitude	✓	✓	✓	✓	✓	✓	✓	✗
Change in behaviour	✓	✓	✓	✓	✓	✓	✓	✗
Change in health	✓	✓	✓	✓	✓	✓	✓	✗
Changes in service	✗	✓	✓	✓	✓	✓	✓	✗
Changes in society	✗	✓	✓	✓	✓	✓	✓	✗

- *Input evaluation* measures whether the programme is being carried out in the expected way. It looks at the broad structure behind the programme; what is being put into it in terms of the quality and quantity of the facilities available, the details of the personnel involved in the delivery of the activity and the details of the recipients.
- *Process evaluation* looks at the implementation and maintenance of the activity. It studies the technique(s) used to share information, content and the response of the recipients.
- *Output evaluation* is concerned with qualitative data which can be produced as a result of the activity; for instance measures taken may include the number of people who use the service, or the number of contacts recipients have with health professionals. Output evaluation can also be manipulated to give data on efficiency of the activity – for instance cost effectiveness.
- *Impact, or outcome evaluation* assesses the effect the activity has on the recipients' knowledge, attitudes, behaviour and long-term health. It tends to be the real test of whether the initial aims and objectives have been achieved. Data collected tends to be of a quantitative nature. As well as measuring the effect of the activity on the recipients, health service and societal changes may also be studied.

The more levels are tested in an evaluation, the broader the total evaluation will be. However, a broad evaluation will not be necessary in all cases (even though it may be desirable, it may not be possible because of limited resources). A midwife may easily be able to monitor or evaluate a parent education course she runs by observing her own reactions and those of participants, and asking for people's assessment of the course, but without the backing of her managers and adequate resources it would be near impossible to effectively test the changes parent education classes make to the quality of parenting in the longer term. Many evaluations deal with short-term impact and outcome, especially of a qualitative nature, but long-term results, especially of a quantitative nature, are much more difficult to follow up.

Although by no means an exhaustive list of the techniques which can be employed to evaluate health promotion, the ones given in Table 7.2 give a range which can measure both qualitative and quantitative consequences.

Interview

The interview is valuable in obtaining information in order to evaluate small-scale health promotion activities and can be a useful tool for larger studies when there are adequate resources to fund the interviewing of a wide range of recipients. Good interviewing allows for ideas to be explored and is particularly useful in collecting qualitative data, for instance whether facilities are felt to be adequate, or whether the content of an activity was appropriate. Its weakness is that some people are not able to be critical when interviewed and may therefore compliment an activity that they did not really feel was useful, or claim to have changed an attitude or behaviour in order to impress the interviewer, especially if the interviewer is known to them as having a keen interest in health. Depending on who is evaluating the activity, both recipients and health promoters, managers or other interested parties may be interviewed to fill in a picture about the activity. Interviewing each person on more than one occasion over a period of time may elicit changes in knowledge, attitudes, behaviour and health status. Such information is of particular interest in evaluating health promotion.

Questionnaire

Questionnaires are used to elicit similar information to that gained by interview, that is qualitative material, often on a larger scale as the interviewer's time is not called upon. However producing a good questionnaire, with straightforward non-contradictory questions can be very difficult. Questionnaires can include attitude/ratings scales (see below), open and closed questions, knowledge questions and other formats which will produce an expanse of information about the activity.

Survey

A survey is, in effect, a large-scale questionnaire which is circulated to many people, so that statistics or quantitative data can be gleaned from the results. Due to the size of the population surveyed, the results are often generalized for similar populations. It is a useful evaluation tool when resources are available to contact and follow up a large sample.

Ratings scale

Ratings scales ask particularly for people's opinions and are useful in asking about the quality of facilities and techniques used and in measuring attitudes. They give easily categorized results, as the respondent may be asked to concur with one of five answers in response to a statement or question; typically, strongly agree, agree, don't know, disagree, strongly disagree (in the case of the Likert Scale), or rank order their opinion of a range of possible choices (as in a Guttman Scale). Space for extra comments in between scales can give a further dimension to the information obtained but are time consuming to analyse where the sample size is large, and comments often confuse the answers given in the scales, rather than add enlightenment for the evaluator.

Focus group

The focus group is a small group of participants who reflect together on a given subject area. Their conversation can provide interesting data for the evaluator on attitudes about input and process, and knowledge and attitudes in outcome. A focus group reconvened some time after the health promotion activity may also give information on long-term impact, as they will between them have a range of beliefs and attitudes. The data available are purely qualitative, as a focus group is by definition small enough for every voice to be heard. Typically a focus group will be used to find out what the going concerns of the group are, so these concerns can provide the basis of what the evaluator measures in the larger group of participants in an activity or programme.

Diary

Diary-keeping is an evaluative technique whereby the activity leaders and/or the participants keep a personal record of how their involvement felt. Again a purely qualitative technique, the information gained gives a picture which the evaluator can use to analyse changes in beliefs and attitudes, reactions to the environment or gain insight into what it feels like to be a part of the activity.

Performance indicators

Performance indicators are a relatively cheap and easy way of measuring end results of health promoting activities, especially impact. As the name suggests, targets by which to measure success are made explicit (for instance 90% of new mothers who start breastfeeding will still be doing so 6 weeks after the birth) and actual figures are collected and compared (*see* Table 7.3). The data collected are quantitative and do not concern process – in effect, the means justify the ends, although it would be foolish of anyone involved in setting performance indicators and collating statistics not to ensure that the systems and resources are in place so that the targets are realistically attainable. While providing valuable widescale statistics on behaviour, performance indicators ignore the emotional and social aspects of health promotion activity and place value on behaviour change, regardless of personal cost. They are the evaluative technique of choice for the government's *Health of the nation* targets for the year 2000 (Department of Health, 1992).

Cost effectiveness studies

Cost effectiveness studies or cost utility studies attempt to weigh up the likely costs and benefits of the activity. Nowadays they usually include a judgement on the value and costs to the woman and families involved, although it is undeniably difficult to quantify women's experiences and decide how they should rate against cost implications for a Health Trust or Authority. Cost effectiveness studies have largely superseded cost benefit analyses which, according to Roberts (1996), tried and not surprisingly largely failed to find a simple formula as to how health promotion resource funding should be spent to benefit everyone.

However, one of the more popular forms of cost benefit analysis which has attempted to evaluate health care need and provision has been made through the calculation of quality-adjusted life years, or QALYs. These received much attention in the 1980s and still generate interest among some health economists. While the common example of QALYs given is the calculation of the number of quality life years following X number of hip replacements versus the quality of life years following X number of heart transplants, a similar calculation could be used when anticipating cost benefits of providing maternity facilities, for instance resources put into the prevention of preterm birth versus resources allocated to neonatal intensive care facilities. The quality of life and number of years lived by surviving babies following preterm birth would form part of this calculation. However Jones and Prowle (1987:161) suggest that QALYs represent

Table 7.3 Setting up and using a performance indicator

Target: 90% of new mothers who start breastfeeding will still be doing so 6 weeks after the birth.
(Suggestions in italics are activities involved around the use of the performance indicator, not part of the evaluation itself.)

1. *Encourage women to breastfeed by positive information-sharing at antenatal appointments, in parent education and throughout the maternity services by baby friendly initiatives and education of maternity staff. (If a Trust or Health Authority adopt positive values about breastfeeding there is a moral duty to make these explicit before performance indicators are put in place and data collected.)*

2. Collect data on number of women who commence breastfeeding at their baby's birth.

3. *Provide support systems for mothers and midwives that enable continuing breastfeeding. (Again, the Trust or Health Authority have a moral duty to champion their own cause – that of sustained breastfeeding.)*

4. Collect data on number of women breastfeeding at 6 weeks postpartum. It would also be useful to collect data of the reasons why women who discontinued breastfeeding during this time, did so, in case the target is not met.

5. Compare breastfeeding rates at birth and at 6 weeks postpartum, and statistically calculate whether the 90% target has been reached or not.

6. Consider the implications of the results and replan for future evaluation.

'a cloak of pseudo-scientific empiricism for what are essentially political decisions' (i.e. their calculation constitutes an unscientific experiment, which attempts to excuse the necessary politico-economic decisions from being made, on which the well-being of the health services depend). While their suggestions for deciding the allocation of resources, listed below, are based on their approach to cost benefit analysis, it is equally relevant in terms of cost effectiveness studies:

1. Priorities and objectives within the Trust or Health Authority are identified.
2. Constraints such as finance or manpower are identified.
3. Alternatives to the present system are generated in the light of the information in 1 and 2.
4. Both capital (i.e. lump sum required to set up an initiative) and running costs are forecast for the costs and savings of each alternative.
5. Financial costs are calculated to give a comparable rate for each alternative.
6. The benefits of each alternative are identified and quantified where possible, not only in monetary terms.
7. Any non-financial social costs are identified.
8. The relevant information on each alternative is presented to the decision-maker.
9. The decision-maker makes an explicit subjective decision about which alternative(s) to implement.
10. Some time after implementation, the success or failure of the investment is reviewed.

Choosing an evaluation technique

The choice of evaluation technique will depend upon a number of factors. Perhaps the most important is, who evaluates. Large organizations have more power and resources to consider sophisticated and widespread evaluation, whereas individuals or small professional groups of individuals have less 'clout' and less resources both in terms of time and finance.

What is being evaluated will also influence the technique. One midwife evaluating her own parent education group may wish to review just one aspect of her own performance, for instance how she facilitates the class. Alternatively she may have a number of evaluation goals, to include not only her own performance, but also the impact of her classes on participants' knowledge or labour/parenting experience, or other factors. She may choose to interview or give questionnaires to all or a representative selection of participants, or she may keep a reflective diary herself or ask participants to do so, or choose some other technique, perhaps not described here.

EXERCISE 7.1   Which evaluation technique?

For each of the three examples below, consider what objectives you would wish to achieve and select as many evaluation techniques as are appropriate, which could test whether or not those objectives have been achieved.

1. A programme of parent education classes.
2. A health authority's attempt to raise long-term breastfeeding rates, specifically by the support it gives to pregnant and newly delivered women.
3. A national campaign to encourage periconception folic acid dietary supplementation in women.

EXERCISE 7.2   Preparing for evaluation

What information and statistics would it be useful to collect while planning a regional approach to reducing the incidence of teenage pregnancy, with a view to producing quantitative evaluative data in 5 years' time?

EXERCISE 7.3   Specific small study evaluation

Design a small study to evaluate the nutrition of pregnant women in an antenatal clinic before and after the introduction of a specialist midwife to advise on dietary matters.

If a health trust evaluates a health promotional activity, the members involved will choose a technique or techniques that are felt best suited to that activity, and likewise for a national evaluation, within the resources allocated for that particular task.

The timing of the evaluation may mean that it is performed while the activity is in progress, or after it has been completed. Again, certain techniques will be suited to ongoing evaluation, and others to a final assessment.

Overall, the most important aspect of evaluation is that the method or methods chosen measure what needs to be measured – whether this is how far the aims and objectives of the activity have been met by studying the input, process, output and/or outcomes, or whether a midwife wishes to monitor or evaluate her own effectiveness in the delivery of the activity by her own or other people's estimation.

However, both altruistic and less benign reasons abound for performing evaluation, and political and non-objective reasoning sometimes surfaces when evaluation methods are chosen. DeBella *et al.* (1986) consider manifest and latent functions of evaluation; manifest considerations being to improve the quality of current programmes and make resource allocation decisions, and latent functions being to use one's power or prestige to control activities or to terminate programmes. Obviously health promotion activities have vested interests for a number of different people, and where the evaluator has a personal interest in the activity, if for instance she has set it up or runs it, she will want it to evaluate well. An outsider overseeing the evaluation is likely to be more objective, but if the purpose of the evaluation is to improve the system, then the recommendations may be less easy for those with vested interests to accept.

Ethical issues in evaluating health promoting activities

There are a number of ethical issues here that deserve consideration. The first is, whose interests does the evaluation serve? The politics of vested interests in choosing an evaluation technique have been discussed briefly earlier in this chapter. The issue of who receives the findings, and what they do with them is also pertinent.

Evaluation can be time-consuming for recipients and frustrating if they do not see any change as a result of the comments they give. Although future recipients may benefit from previous evaluations if the information gained was made use of, they will not if the evaluator has not done anything with their findings. This often happens if the evaluation gives information which is difficult to interpret because the aims of the activity were not clearly thought out at the beginning and the evaluations give such a wide range of feedback that it is impossible to decide whether the activity was indeed effective, and how it could be improved.

Given that evaluation has been reasonably well carried out and conclusions drawn, decisions must be made about who holds responsibility for incorporating the findings in future practice. If the conclusions recommend the investment of further resources, it may be impossible for the non-budget-holding evaluator to act.

The inconvenience of any evaluation should be considered and weighed up against the value of the information that it provides. While *not* evaluating health promotional activities has major and obvious ethical dimensions, to evaluate must also be viewed in an ethical context.

Summary of key points

- It is important that health promotion interventions are evaluated in terms of health effectiveness and cost effectiveness. A systematic approach to evaluation, starting with clear, realistic, measurable objectives can go far in further enhancing the interventions and activities on offer for childbearing women.

- Evaluation usually involves two processes; first, measuring the activity undertaken, and secondly, comparing it against an agreed standard. Where the second process is not followed, 'monitoring' is a more accurate description, although such monitoring is frequently described as evaluation in the literature.
- Evaluation may be qualitative or quantitative, and often both types are used because each renders important information. Qualitative and quantitative data gained on the same activity can also complement each other well in terms of demonstrating its effectiveness (or otherwise) from different angles.
- As well as helping midwives and other health workers to know what they are doing well and where a system could be improved, evaluation is needed to ensure that in areas of finite resources, money is being efficiently invested in effective health promotion activities and programmes.
- Evaluation, and acting on the information gained to improve the process and outcomes, should be built in to all activities and programmes as an ongoing process, as with planning, thereby making evaluation a continuous dynamic, rather than a one-off activity.
- The effectiveness of health promotion to date is largely unknown because many projects are embarked upon with no evaluation plan, with assumptions being made about unquestioned benefit.
- The commonest reasons for lack of evaluation are the time and resources it can consume, the cost of which may not have been built in at the planning stage, and fear of the process, seen by many as unduly difficult and complicated.
- Techniques used in the evaluation process include interviewing, questionnaires, surveys, ratings scales, focus groups, diary-keeping, performance indicators and cost effectiveness studies. The technique(s) used will depend upon what is being evaluated, and by whom. Time and resources must also be considered.
- There are always vested and political interests involved in evaluation. There will be people who believe that an activity should continue because they have invested personal resources in it (and who will design an evaluation to reflect this), and those whose interest lies in their own interpretation of cost effectiveness. The interests of the people whom the activity or intervention is designed to help can often be misplaced by the personal politics of organizers and managers.

References

DeBella, S., Martin, L. and Siddall, S. 1986: *Nurses' role in health care planning.* Connecticut: Appleton-Century-Crofts.

Department of Health 1992: *The health of the nation: a strategy for health in England.* London: HMSO.

Downie, R.S., Fyfe, C. and Tannahill, A. 1996: *Health promotion models and values.* Oxford: Oxford University Press.

Hawe, P., Degeling, D. and Hall, J. 1990: *Evaluating health promotion.* Artarmon, NSW, Australia: MacLennan and Petty.

Health Education Authority 1994: *Helping pregnant smokers quit: training for health professionals.* London: Health Education Authority.

Jones, T. and Prowle, M. 1987: *Health service finance: an introduction.* London: The Certified Accountants Educational Trust.

Roberts, J. 1996: Changing childbirth – choices and costs. *MIDIRS Midwifery Digest* 6(3), 261–63.

Further reading

Bunton, R. and Macdonald, G. (eds) 1992: *Health promotion disciplines and diversities.* London: Routledge.

Connor, A. 1993: *Monitoring and evaluation made easy – a handbook for voluntary organisations.* Edinburgh: HMSO.

Ewles, L. and Simnett, I. 1995: *Promoting health.* London: Scutari Press.

Part II

Interpersonal skills: the cornerstone of effective health promotion

8

Midwives and communication

Studies in childbirth that examine women's satisfaction levels demonstrate the need for midwives to be constantly aware of the effect of communication, both good and bad, at such a sensitive time. Good communication leads to greater satisfaction for both mothers and midwives, and studies such as the triennial Department of Health reports into maternal mortality clearly demonstrate that effective communication also underpins safe practice.

This chapter will cover two themes. The first will consider what constitutes good communication, and the second will evaluate what midwifery research teaches us about the ways we communicate in our practice. While acknowledging the importance of interdisciplinary communication, this chapter will deal with the issue of effective communication between mothers and midwives in promoting health.

What is good communication?

Although it is often easy to look at a given interaction between people and decide whether or not they communicated effectively, it is much harder to try to define what constitutes good communication. Getting the message across is obviously important, but so too is the way people feel about the message (particularly if the information is not that which they wish to hear), how long information is retained, and a host of other issues, some personal and some general.

Yet it seems that it is impossible to get this aspect of practice exactly right – improvement is something that must constantly be striven for. In recent years there has been growing midwifery and sociological research on how midwives communicate, especially on what women appreciate, and what they would like more of, in terms of communication with midwives and other health professionals.

A good way to interpret what constitutes effective communication is to examine communication models, which rather than attempt a unidimensional definition, give a broader picture of what human interaction entails. In Fig. 8.1 the ideas of Gerard Egan (1994) are incorporated into a diagram or simple model comprising the basic skills required in order to communicate effectively.

Perceptiveness of what goes on in any interaction or series of interactions is crucial to good communication to make it sensitive and effective. The type of communication that involves 'lecturing' or 'preaching' has rightly received a bad press in professional practice and has no place in adult communication – it shows lack of perceptiveness of both the need for mutual non-judgemental respect, and the sensitivity required to leave a positive memory of the interaction for both parties. Heightened self-

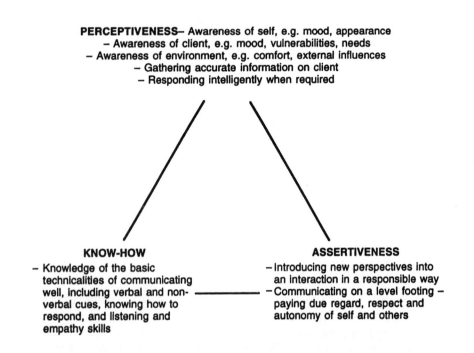

PERCEPTIVENESS– Awareness of self, e.g. mood, appearance
– Awareness of client, e.g. mood, vulnerabilities, needs
– Awareness of environment, e.g. comfort, external influences
– Gathering accurate information on client
– Responding intelligently when required

KNOW-HOW
– Knowledge of the basic technicalities of communicating well, including verbal and non-verbal cues, knowing how to respond, and listening and empathy skills

ASSERTIVENESS
– Introducing new perspectives into an interaction in a responsible way
– Communicating on a level footing – paying due regard, respect and autonomy of self and others

Figure 8.1 Aspects of communication (Adapted from Egan, 1994)

awareness and awareness of the perspectives of others will enhance effective communication. The concept of reflection helps us to observe ourselves and our actions, and ask ourselves if we would react to a situation in the same way again, or whether there is room for improvement. Maturity in acknowledging our own mistakes will enhance both perceptiveness and improvement in communication skills. Perceptiveness develops through experience.

Know-how involves both understanding the communication process and the ability to deliver appropriate responses. Understanding the role and presence of verbal and non-verbal cues and messages given both consciously and unconsciously to the other parties, and listening and empathy skills are important. Like perceptiveness, know-how improves with experience in professional encounters. It also depends upon a certain amount of self-confidence which can develop from self-awareness. Know-how will help the midwife to understand the underlying, as well as the overt messages in an interaction, so she can help people to articulate information and feelings that may otherwise be left unsaid, or said in a way that masks their true import and meaning. However the midwife also needs to consider respecting the privacy of the other person in not wishing to reveal certain information. Her subtle technical abilities will allow her the intuition to know when to encourage self-revelation, and when to heed privacy.

Assertiveness is important to good communication because it acknowledges the necessity for equality in the relationships between the participants, and the autonomy of each – the right to make one's own decisions, regardless of the opinions of others, and the right to make mistakes.

There are many other communication models in existence, putting different stresses on different aspects of communicating in human relationships. Egan is interested in the helping relationship set up by professional counsellors, making his work particularly relevant to midwives.

The qualities of a skilled communicator

Effective communication ultimately liberates people, helping them in various ways to find new depths in themselves and new meanings about the world around them. Good communication should leave people feeling better about themselves because they have been listened to, given and received information, shared a joke or perhaps expressive eye contact. Even criticism can be good communication when offered tactfully and for the right reasons – it can help to develop self-awareness and improvement in understanding. There are a number of qualities that skilled communicators possess; some of these are listed below.

Genuineness

Genuineness is one of the most important qualities in interpersonal relationships. There is no façade and the woman knows she is dealing with a 'real' person, so games and ploys are not necessary – personally meaningful communication can take place.

Empathy

Empathy means taking seriously the ideas, beliefs and concerns of the other party. It is the ability to put oneself in another person's position, and see things from her perspective.

Kindness

It seems rather obvious to state kindness, but it is a skill many women isolate as crucial to the skills of a midwife, and complain about if they see it as lacking. Small acts of kindness are often remembered for a long time, as are perceived acts of unkindness.

Respect

Communication is rarely effective without respect being overtly shown. This incorporates acceptance of the woman for what she is unconditionally and without judgement of her *person*, although the midwife may see it as her role to express judgement on health *habits*, such as smoking or intention to breast- or bottle-feed. Psychologist Carl Rogers describes positive regard of the person as an effective enhancer of interpersonal communication.

Honesty

Again, honesty may seem a fairly obvious component of effective communication but it can be difficult in some situations for a health professional to say 'I don't know' or 'I was wrong', when they feel this may lower their status in the eyes of the woman. However most people value honesty as it engenders trust – no one can be expected to know everything, and no one is right all of the time. It can often be valuable for individuals, especially health professionals, to show their vulnerability without loss of face – it makes them more human and may help the woman to value her own knowledge and responsibility more highly. In many situations honesty requires confidence and courage, especially when it is thought likely to raise the anxiety of the woman. Dishonesty or concealment of information is usually discovered fairly quickly, and this can have long-term serious consequences for the woman in her dealings with all health professionals who have future contact with her.

Diplomacy

Diplomacy is necessary for skilled communication, especially when there is bad news to impart. It can prepare the woman and prevent unnecessary anxiety (although it should not prevent all anxiety if this is a suitable reaction to a situation). Again, it is a skill that develops with experience, often of previously poorly managed situations, and practice.

Developing rapport

This is the ability to make people feel comfortable and able to 'open up'. Health professionals, by the nature of their relationships with others, are required to be able to develop rapport very quickly, none more so than the midwife who meets a woman or couple for the first time during the woman's labour.

Self-awareness

Burnard (1986:15) describes self-awareness as 'the gradual and continuous process of noticing and exploring aspects of the self, whether behavioural, psychological or physical, with the intention of developing personal and interpersonal understanding. Such awareness cannot be developed for its own sake; it is intimately bound up with our relationship with others', and he continues, 'to become more aware of, and to have a deeper understanding of ourselves is to have a sharper and clearer picture of what is happening to others.' Burnard also differentiates between self-awareness and self-consciousness, self-consciousness being a state of being painfully aware of ourselves, which is often very obvious to others. Self-consciousness is therefore not helpful in developing self-awareness and can impede it.

Reflection

Once self-awareness starts to take place, reflection can develop. By reflecting on one's practice, knowledge and experience can be transformed into personal and meaningful learning strategies, and knowledge and practice developed to make them dynamic forces, moving away from routine, unquestioning dogma. Education and professional care become more of a partnership between teacher and learner, midwife and mother; creativity and personal autonomy are enhanced and from this inspiration develops.

Balancing skills

A knack of communicating well is to be able to balance when to listen, when to provide information and when to offer advice. Sometimes women will desire only unbiased information, or sometimes support for a decision they have come to having weighed up the evidence available for themselves. Sometimes they will wish for advice. It is a real skill, borne out of awareness, to differentiate and react to different needs at different times.

Standing back

Once again, standing back from a situation is a skill developed through self-awareness and experience. It allows the woman to make her choice and live with it, and respects her for her right to choose. For the midwife it means not being personally affronted if a woman chooses to continue to smoke, or partake in health-damaging behaviour, but continuing to provide support which is non-judgemental of the person.

Different aspects of communication

It is useful to clarify some of the language used when discussing modes of communication because the increasing sophistication of communication studies is revealing. Information-giving, information-sharing, counselling and counselling skills each have their role to play but are suitable for different aspects of interactions, although all may be required within the same conversation. Often the most straightforward conversations that midwives have can be misinterpreted because there is confusion in matching the information to be shared with the mode in which it can best be aired. Some differentiation is offered here of the following inter-actions.

Information-giving and information-sharing

Information-giving should be offered in as unbiased a way as possible. However it is practically impossible to do this without attaching, some-times quite subconsciously, our own values. The most obvious example is highlighting the information we actually do share with each woman; bearing in mind we cannot share everything, we choose to share what *we* think she needs to know. The order in which she is given a variety of information, say on nutrition, perhaps says more about what the midwife thinks is important about a good diet than anything else. However careful the midwife is in trying to suppress the expression of her personal values, some will always come through and this can leave the woman to sort out the issues important to her from those important to someone else. Making one's own opinion known can also reduce the effectiveness of the message. If, in imparting information on fetal screening tests the midwife states 'I think it is a very good idea for all women over the age of forty to have an amniocentesis', the woman has not only the risk ratio to consider, but also the issue of whether or not she should be influenced by a health professional with perhaps superior knowledge of the physical aspects of the test, but far less awareness of the woman's attitudes to screening, abortion, children with disabilities and the host of other issues involved.

Although information-giving is sometimes valuable, information-*sharing* in many cases may be more appropriate – and the midwife being honest with herself and the woman about her own views (when these are sought). Encouraging the woman to develop her own thoughts may be one of the most valuable issues aired. The midwife may encourage information-sharing by opening the discussion with 'How do you feel about the tests available in pregnancy to look for problems with the baby?' or 'Is there any information you need about screening tests to look for problems with the baby in pregnancy?' For women not able to think of any questions at this point some further cues may be useful, such as 'Had you thought of having any of the tests?'. Although information-giving is likely to form a large part of the conversation on the subject of screening tests, this should not be done without some sharing of the woman's feelings and previous knowledge, as great offence may be caused if attitudes to such issues as abortion are ignored. Women will also feel more valued if their thoughts and experience are given importance by the midwife. The assertiveness issue is also pertinent here in each party feeling comfortable in rejecting the other's perceived values if they do not suit their own.

Checking understanding

In some situations the midwife may feel it is important to check that information given or shared has been correctly understood by both sides. She can do this in a number of ways. Perhaps the least effective is to repeat her interpretation of it, although this will not necessarily be unhelpful. She may discuss the information with the woman, taking care to listen for understanding being demonstrated in interpreting the information. Alternatively she may ask the woman to repeat the information, taking care not to do so in a patronizing way.

Advising

Information-giving and advising are often confused, partly because they frequently occur together. With the development of partnership in care between woman and midwife and reflective practice the actual custom of giving advice should decrease, because it presupposes that it is helpful for midwives to interpret information for women rather than allow women to do so for themselves. Of course, women often ask for advice (sometimes confusing it themselves with a request for information) and sometimes it is appropriate to advise – for instance, it would be appropriate for a midwife to advise a woman to seek immediate midwifery or medical attention if she describes symptoms of pre-eclampsia over the telephone. However in some situations advice-giving is inappropriate. A woman complaining of early pregnancy nausea and vomiting is likely to be better helped by discussing a range of coping strategies involving diet and eating habits, rest, exercise, coping with nausea when at work, etc. than being advised to adopt one or two methods of dealing with the situation. Better still, if she is encouraged to explore her own ideas and experiences of coping strategies, she is more likely to feel confident and self-reliant in her own resources, and deal more confidently with future personal inconveniences. She will also perceive that the midwife has confidence in her ability to do so.

Counselling and using counselling skills

Counselling is another mode of interpersonal communication which is also often grossly misunderstood. 'She was counselled to have the test' and 'the purpose of the counselling was to help them get over their bereavement' are examples of such misunderstanding – counselling is necessarily much more open-ended than this. Counselling may help a person to explore the issues to decide whether or not she wishes to have an antenatal screening test; it may help a couple to express their feelings about their dead baby, but it will never dictate to them how they feel, or how they should feel, about that loss. Midwives may frequently employ counselling skills in an interaction (for instance listening attentively, empathizing, providing verbal and non-verbal cues and responding appropriately) but most will not act as a 'counsellor' as such in their day-to-day practice. Counselling is necessarily time-consuming when done effectively, and requires a great deal of personal preparation, and some would say years of study and practice in its own right. The counsellor and the person and people with whom he or she gives counsel usually enter into a contract together, often informally but in which they agree the nature of the problem and how it should be tackled.

Supporting

Supporting is listed here as a communication skill important to midwives because it is mentioned so often in ward handovers and in relation to women with difficult pregnancies. However its true meaning gains little space in textbooks and learning materials. It is commonly mentioned in research study conclusions as what women say they want as a priority from midwives, especially when experiencing difficulties with their health or their encounters with the health services. Support in this context means positively to encourage, for instance with a woman in labour or breastfeeding; to provide and share information, for instance about antenatal facilities and benefits available and early postnatal care of the newborn; and advocacy in some circumstances, for instance when ensuring that the stated wishes on a birthplan are carried out when the woman is unable to hold a conversation while in strong labour. Support may also be of a physical nature, for instance helping a woman to get to and from the bathroom, tidy her bed or pass her her baby in the early days following a Caesarean section when she is in pain and has no visitors present to help. By definition it is the woman or couple who are the final judges of whether effective support has been given following the event.

Communication barriers

We all come across blocks in communication in our day-to-day lives, possibly as frequently as we encounter effective skills in use. Understanding why they happen can help to reduce them. Some common barriers include the following.

Stress

Reduced resources, shortages of staff, poor motivation, tiredness after a long shift and personal problems at home can all lead to increased stress and a block in communication due to lack of time to explain and discuss, an abrupt exchange or avoidance of an interaction altogether. Poor self-esteem may be a precursor or result of stress and a midwife or mother who does not value herself will have difficulty in communicating with others effectively.

Personality clash

Sometimes people find that they cannot communicate with each other and don't even like to share company. This can be difficult if they are expected to work together in a team, and solutions often depend upon the maturity of both parties to tackle their differences.

Clashes of personality are likely to become a more widespread problem with caseload practice where midwives are required to work very closely with each other and the same pregnant women over a fairly long period of time. Although a difficult problem to address and deal with, the availability of intermediaries and systems where midwives and women can change their relationships with a minimum of hassle, and further support systems to help people to deal with the clash and subsequent rejection may be helpful but inevitably time-consuming.

Social and cultural differences

Different languages, cultural backgrounds, values and beliefs are well-documented barriers to communication. Patience, tolerance and genuine respect for the other party are crucial to prevent prejudicial encounters, although such differences between people of different race, creed and ethnic background, etc. require much deeper understanding and action to eradicate the barriers. These problems are further addressed in the later section of this chapter 'Midwives, research and communication'. Openness to accept different backgrounds and ideas on both sides will help towards removing the barriers.

Limited information/understanding/memory

Depth of communication will be lost if any or all of these are lacking. The use of jargon is also detrimental to good communication. Everyday phrases used by midwives such as 'membrane rupture', 'contractions' (perhaps only known as labour pains to some women) or 'fetal abnormality' (birthmarks? brain damage?) may cause confusion to the woman who may never have heard the expression before. I include below three examples I have seen in practice of limited understanding of midwifery language, all by women whose first language was English.

Situation 1

Midwife:	Have you thought about whether you would like to breast- or bottlefeed?
Pregnant woman:	Yes, bottlefeed. I saw a TV programme last night which said that breastfeeding was very unhealthy.
Midwife:	I missed that. It sounds interesting. Why is breastfeeding unhealthy?
Pregnant woman:	It must cause heart attacks in later life, because for the first few days the baby gets pure cholesterol.
Midwife:	I wonder if you are confusing cholesterol and colostrum?

Situation 2

The midwife explains to a woman in labour that her baby is distressed, and she wishes to call in the duty doctor to see the heart trace. The woman promptly bursts into tears. When gently asked why, she replies that she had no idea that an unborn baby could get upset and cry.

Situation 3

A woman, 16 weeks pregnant, is adamant that she does not want an alpha-fetoprotein test. She explains that she has been informed about the test by another midwife – that it is to check for spina bifida and other neural tube defects, but is not 100 per cent accurate, that the results take a few days and that if the baby is found to be abnormal she will have the opportunity to discuss termination of pregnancy. She seems to be very knowledgeable, which the midwife comments on. The woman then adds, 'I know most women do opt to have this test, but I just don't know how they can bear that needle through their tummy.'

As well as medical jargon, colloquial language can also cause problems in understanding for women from other parts of the English-speaking world, as well as those for whom English is not a first language. Pain, anxiety, anger and many other conditions and distractions can affect understanding and memory.

Contradictory or inconsistent advice

This is a frequent complaint of both mothers and midwives. Consistency depends to a large extent on effective sharing of information, beliefs and values. Coming to a consensus of opinion based on available evidence can take hours of debate and discussion, and is often not reached despite the needs of an organization to project shared ideas and principles. Contradictory expressed ideas of one individual can throw a whole team into disarray and utterly confuse outsiders. This happens with government dissenters as well as within organizations such as the NHS! However it can cause major disharmony and confusion to such groups as breastfeeding mothers. The results in such a case, as we have seen in the UK, are low uptake rates and early discontinuation of breastfeeding.

Inconsistencies are also seen when official advice changes or the experts disagree, for instance on the value of HIV antibody testing, or routine Caesarean section for all babies presenting by the breech.

Midwives, research and communication

Research into the ways midwives communicate can be broadly arranged into a number of different approaches:

1. research that seeks out women's views;
2. observational studies of midwives at work;
3. the research on the indirect effect of communication, on such primary issues as successful breastfeeding, satisfaction rates with maternity care, etc.; and
4. studies on the usefulness of interventions to enhance communication such as written information, leaflets and parent education aids.

This section reports on a number of recent research projects into mid-wives' communication skills, and how we may use these to develop and enhance good practice.

Such research reveals a wealth of data which can inform us about what women want (and don't want) from midwives. It can tell us about women from different backgrounds and cultures. We can learn and become more aware of the more subtle responses of midwives and women to each other, and it can inform us about the similarities and differences in needs and expectations of women and midwives.

The research studies quoted in this chapter on communication in the antenatal, labour and postnatal periods are by no means an exhaustive coverage of all the studies done, but are chosen to illustrate how research can be utilized to make us all think about and further develop our own skills. However it should be remembered that research cannot tell us how to respond in individual situations requiring good and effective commu-nication – it may guide us, but the woman's wishes, commonsense and experience will be equally valuable in deciding a best course of action.

Communication in the antenatal period

In a study of mothers' views about information and advice in pregnancy and birth, Ann Jacoby in 1988 received questionnaires from 1508 women, completed approximately 4 months after the births of their babies, from ten areas of England. She discovered that although women were satisfied on the whole with the information and advice that they were given during pregnancy, a fifth would have liked more information, yet felt unable to discuss issues with midwives as fully as they would have liked. Interestingly, a further fifth felt that they were given too much informa-tion about some things, and not enough about others. Of the 628 primigravidae, 43 per cent had discussed the process of childbirth with a midwife or nurse, yet reading was the most frequently mentioned source of information, by 78 per cent of the women.

Jacoby asked the women whether during their pregnancy they had been able fully to discuss the things they wanted with doctors, midwives and nurses. Twenty-four per cent felt unable to do so and Jacoby found these feelings were related to their social class, marital status and housing tenure, but not to their parity or ethnic origin. The unmarried, those of manual social class and those who did not own their own home felt unable to discuss things fully. The higher the social class, the more likely the woman was to have discussed birth issues, and valued the informa-tion given.

Jacoby's discovery that Asian women were more likely to say that they had the right amount of information came as a surprise, given language and cultural differences. The explanations of this factor are varied; Asian women were underrepresented in the sample, and may also have been less likely to return their questionnaires. They may also have been more accepting than questioning of information presented to them due to their cultural background, especially of health professionals, often male, who were seen as in authority.

A more detailed analysis of the communication problems of women of Asian descent comes from Isobel Bowler (1993). Using a theme of communication problems, she observed the stereotypes that midwives used in order to 'classify' women and organize care. In her study, which observed Asian women's interactions with midwives, she found that the women were often shy about their customs and limited understanding of the English language, and were therefore classified by midwives as rude, unresponsive and/or unintelligent. For instance, midwives felt that the women did not say 'please' or 'thank you' and often gave orders. However in Urdu such words are often not said, but implied by a form of the imperative with the 'please' being built into the verb. Therefore the women did not intend to be rude, but were perceived as such by the midwives. Ultimately, Asian women were thought of as 'bad' patients, and the stereotypes which the midwives built up reinforced these negative views of the women. Bowler concluded that midwives can be sympathetic yet still stereotype; that stereotypes in this situation are inevitably racist; and that until cultural barriers can be broken down and individualized care offered to all women, midwifery communication will suffer.

The communication of information about fetal screening tests in pregnancy is also receiving increasing research interest, which culminated in the Informed Choice leaflets 'Looking for Down's syndrome and spina bifida in pregnancy' and 'Antenatal screening for congenital abnormalities: helping women to choose' produced by MIDIRS and the NHS Centre for Reviews and Dissemination in 1997. One of the problems of communicating such information for midwives is that it is complicated and necessarily time-consuming. There may be confusion about the difference between a screening and a diagnostic test, and the nature of individual experiences of conditions such as spina bifida and Down's syndrome are impossible to predict, thereby causing further difficulty in helping women and couples to form an accurate picture of how their child born with such a condition may affect their lives.

In order to avoid addressing some of these complicated issues, midwives will often concentrate on the physical aspects of screening tests and either side-step or give limited time to discussion about the social and psychological consequences. Women may however be left feeling very cheated of professional support if doubt is raised about the well-being of their pregnancy but emotional support and information are lacking.

The literature stresses the importance of midwives and health professionals exploring their own values and beliefs as a prerequisite in

providing non-judgemental information and support. It also acknowledges the need for them to be knowledgeable about fetal screening tests,
and the communication skills necessary to collect and present information
in ways that make women feel informed and supported. Continuing
education which covers communication as well as clinical issues, prefera-
bly addressed together, is seen as vital if midwives are to be effective and
women empowered rather than emotionally injured by the maternity
services.

Communication in the antenatal period can clearly be improved on
many fronts, not just those mentioned here. Jacoby (1988) suggests that in
studies of maternity services poor communication is often due to over-
crowded and busy clinics, staff attitudes and a lack of continuity of care.
She quotes the Association of Community Health Councils in England
and Wales who wrote in 1987: 'the biggest improvements in antenatal care
could be made by changes in administrative and management procedures
and the adoption of a more sympathetic and considerate attitude by
clinical staff and service providers', and concludes that such changes
would do much to improve women's satisfaction with their maternity
care.

Communication in labour

Perhaps the best-known midwifery researcher into communication
between midwives and mothers in labour is Mavis Kirkham. However,
communication during the birth process is becoming an increasingly
researched theme from a number of different angles, which when considered together can give a broader picture of what actually happens
during communication at this time.

Jacoby's (1988) study, which looked at information and advice about
birth as well as pregnancy, found that 79 per cent of her sample felt that
they had received enough information during labour, but around 19 per
cent would have liked more information than they actually got. She
makes the very important point that kindness by the midwife led to
greater satisfaction by women who then perceived that they received
good information.

Kirkham's communication studies have been reported over a number
of years (1983a, b, 1989). She has concentrated on how midwives communicate with women in labour by herself sitting in on labours and writing
observational notes for subsequent analysis. The originality of this
research has led to the development of theories which have far-reaching
consequences for the delivery of midwifery care. Kirkham writes about
how she observed midwives block and deflect questions from women
during labour (1983b), thereby inhibiting future questioning by the
woman. She noticed that women of higher social class asked for and
received more information than women from lower social classes, as

midwives made assumptions about the depth of information such women would understand. Women of lower social class often sought information by humble or passive techniques, for instance by denigrating themselves. Midwives stereotyped women and then gave them the information which they considered appropriate. Kirkham also reported that the involvement of senior staff in a labour had an inhibiting effect on communication offered by a primary midwife.

Kirkham (1989:125) develops Sheila Kitzinger's idea of 'verbal asepsis'. A typical example of such a conversation goes:

Woman: 'How long does it take?'
Sister: 'Babies come when they're ready.'
Woman: (Changes subject).

In such conversations midwives avoid answering questions that they have no answer to, and deflect women's concerns. It also has the effect of preventing the woman from having the information she needs to be involved in decision-making, leaving the professionals in control. 'Routine patter' is also developed by midwives to introduce women to the policies of the labour ward, and block their individuality from being expressed.

Kirkham (1989) also explores the concept of 'reassurance' which midwives so often use to try to allay fear, but she noted in many cases that this ploy simply resembled a denial of the woman's apprehensions, by bland cheer such as 'Don't worry'. This was seen to have the effect of quietening the woman concerned, and making the midwife feel better because she assumed that she had indeed allayed the woman's fears.

Kirkham's research is a key component in helping us to reflect on how what we do and what we say to women in labour can really affect them. She concludes that the use of language is crucial in labour and communication will not improve until language becomes more woman-orientated – not just in terms of jargon, but midwives must also stop blocking and deflecting difficult questions, offering empty reassurances and developing routine patter which negates the individuality of every woman, her labour, and her relationships with her carers.

Hewison (1993) analyses the use of language and terminology in labour and concludes, like Kirkham, that language determines social constructs and midwives must develop language with mothers in order to effect change.

Although McKay and Yager Smith's study, published in 1993, is based on American women's birth experiences, there are some useful findings which relate to women of all backgrounds. Like Kirkham, they found that women want more information and emotional support in labour, but their midwives when interviewed separately thought that they were providing good care and were not aware of any breach between the perceptions of themselves and the women in their care over the quality of their communication. McKay and Yager Smith discovered that the women in their study wanted specific anticipatory information, where possible, on the progress of labour. They did not want false hope when things were not progressing well and they were frequently aware of being given incomplete information. The researchers concluded that information-giving in labour was inadequate in their study, and the process of information-sharing with women in labour must be encouraged and developed; only then will satisfaction rates improve.

Bluff and Holloway in 1994 in the UK examined women's experiences of labour and birth and found a great deal of trust of midwives being expressed by women. However, the women interviewed wanted to be actively involved in decision-making with a flexible approach by their carers. Bluff and Holloway felt that in the past midwives and doctors had encouraged women to hand over responsibility and behave passively in labour (by the means described by Kirkham). They found that where this still occurred, women often did not know how to communicate their needs in labour, and midwives often did not realize that women were so disempowered. They suggest that midwives explore this issue and also whether in reality equality between mother and midwife can be achieved. A great deal of paternalism still exists in maternity care, and health professionals should seek to reduce this wherever possible.

Communication in the postnatal period

Research into communication between mother and midwife in the postnatal period can either be broad or specific, for instance concentrating on issues such as breastfeeding or family planning.

On the theme of the broad issue of postnatal care, Jean Ball has written up her findings of 'the factors that influence the emotional response to motherhood, and to examine the degree to which current patterns of postnatal care given by midwives assist or detract from the adjustment process' (1989:154). Ball measured the influence of midwifery care on the emotional response of the mother to the changes which followed the birth of the baby by questionnaires to the mothers and midwives concerned.

In her sample of 279 women who returned their questionnaire up to 6 weeks postnatally, 109 (39 per cent) complained of conflicting advice from midwives. By comparing a number of variables, and by the nature of her methodology, Ball was able to ascertain that conflicting advice for new mothers was one of a number of factors that contributed to spiralling low self-esteem and emotional distress. The psychological mechanism for this was felt to be that reduced self-confidence induced by conflicting advice led to women blaming themselves and assuming that they were at fault in being unable to breastfeed successfully. Other factors in the way midwives managed postnatal care were seen to enhance or disturb the woman's satisfaction with motherhood; these included encouraging rooming in with the baby in hospital and feeding during the first hour after delivery, which both correlated positively with maternal satisfaction. Ball quotes the psychiatrist Caplan in suggesting that health professionals, and midwives in this case, have the power to 'load the dice' in favour of good or bad emotional outcomes. She suggests a flexible approach in enabling women to adjust and adapt to motherhood whereby provision of encouragement and praise enhance confidence and mental well-being.

Stamp and Crowther (1994), in an Australian study of women's views of their postnatal care by midwives, noted that such studies, concentrating on the time after birth, are few and far between. However, they sent questionnaires shortly after birth and at six weeks postnatally to 235 women, with a 95 per cent response rate. Their results demonstrated midwife helpfulness in hospital related by 74 per cent of the women, and comments made about midwife unhelpfulness in hospital made by 40 per cent of the sample. (Some women commented on both helpful and unhelpful incidences with midwives, hence the overall result totalling more than 100 per cent.) One of the questions the women were asked was 'What was most helpful?' The categories which came out were emotional support; questions answered; information available; information volunteered; help with breastfeeding; help with baby care, and physical care. Emotional support received the greatest number of comments and physical care the least. This distribution of helpfulness was similar shortly after the birth and when the baby was 6 weeks old. Responses to the question about unhelpfulness (most often the first mentioned category) were lack of sensitivity; conflicting advice; judgemental or unsupportive attitudes; insufficient information; too busy – no follow-up; exclusion from decision-making; and inadequate physical care. When asked what would be more helpful from midwives postnatally women most often reported a more supportive attitude. Also high on the list were more flexibility, more information and more consistency. Although a small study and conducted in Australia, where health care administration is vastly different from that in the UK, Stamp and Crowther's findings are likely to have some common threads with British maternity care. Jacoby's 1988 study in England found that 21 per cent of her sample found it rather or very difficult to find out what they wanted to know about their own and their baby's condition, treatment and progress, and 14 per cent found infant feeding advice 'unhelpful'. However in both the above studies some women mentioned that shortage of midwives in the postnatal areas was likely to be a major reason for communication problems.

Lynda Rajan in 1993 commented on a specific and frequently mentioned topic of discussion in midwives' communication as that of breastfeeding support and advice. She quotes Inch and Garforth (1989) who suggest that further research should look at why professional behaviour has remained 'so deeply affected by unfounded assumptions, in spite of the obvious detrimental effect these assumptions have had on breast feeding'. This is an interesting point, although part of the answer is probably obvious – it is far easier for a midwife to offer a bottle of milk or a nipple shield, than help sort out the root cause of sore nipples, engorged breasts or insufficient milk, especially when she is feeling busy and rushed. If the midwife herself is not completely committed to breastfeeding, it will be harder for her to devote her time and energy to helping mothers and babies to succeed in the process.

Rajan discovered that satisfaction with midwifery care during and after the birth was crucial to breastfeeding success. The most commonly expressed needs of the women were for clearer information, non-conflicting advice and practical support during initial attempts at breastfeeding. Many suggested that breastfeeding counsellors should attend the postnatal wards. Rajan suggests that it is necessary for all midwives to be aware of breastfeeding research in order to inform women correctly. Encouragement by midwives was also highly valued by breastfeeding mothers.

Summary of key points

- Good communication both enhances the experience of childbirth for women and their families, and underpins safe practice.
- Definitions of communication often fail to capture the dynamic nature of human interaction. The communication model based on the work of Egan (1994), which explores the dimensions of perceptiveness, know-how and assertiveness more usefully encapsulates the nature of effective professional communication as it affects midwives.
- The qualities of a skilled communicator include genuineness, empathy, kindness, respect for others and self-awareness. Without these and other equally important qualities important messages are lost.
- When possible, information-sharing involving partnership is usually preferable to information-giving. Although the midwife may start with the better knowledge of the facts and figures associated with, for instance, fetal screening tests, the woman's knowledge of her own attitudes towards abortion and disability are an equally important part of any discussion, and should be acknowledged as such.
- Midwives should resist mistaking a request for information as a request for advice. Although advice-giving is sometimes appropriate, a woman who is encouraged to express and develop her own coping strategies is more likely to develop confidence in her own abilities. This will be particularly useful to the new, inexperienced mother.
- Counselling skills, such as listening and empathizing, are useful tools for midwives to possess in enhancing supportive relationships. 'Counselling' as such is a time-consuming, highly skilled process which is

most often performed by a professional counsellor who enters into a contract with the counsellee(s) with agreement as to the nature of the problem and how it is to be tackled.

- Support, in the context of midwifery communication, constitutes positive encouragement, providing and sharing information, and where appropriate, advocacy.
- Common barriers to effective communication include stress, personality clashes, social and cultural differences and limited information or understanding. One of the most commonly quoted communication barriers in the midwifery literature is inconsistent advice.
- Research into the way that midwives communicate tends to concentrate on women's views, observational studies of midwives at work, indirect effects of communication such as the effect on breastfeeding, and the usefulness of interventions, such as leaflets to enhance communication. Such studies offer a wealth of data and theory generation, as well as important implications for improving practice.
- There is always room for improvement in issues such as professional communication and as well as a need for us all to continually develop sensitivity in day-to-day actions, there is a more sophisticated need for the profession of midwifery to consider our language, our routines and the social constructs we place on pregnancy, birth and early parenting with a view to continual improvement.

References

Ball, J. 1989: Postnatal care and adjustment to motherhood. In Robinson, S. and Thomson, A.M. (eds), *Midwives, research and childbirth*, Vol. 1. London: Chapman and Hall, 154–75.

Bluff, R. and Holloway, H. 1994: 'They know best': women's perceptions of midwifery care during labour and childbirth. *Midwifery* 10, 157–64.

Bowler, I.M.W. 1993: Stereotypes of women of Asian descent in midwifery: some evidence. *Midwifery* 9, 7–16.

Burnard, P. 1986: *Learning human skills*. London: Heinemann Medical Books.

Egan, G. 1994: *The skilled helper*. Pacific Grove, California: Brooks/Cole Publishing.

Hewison, A. 1993: The language of labour: an examination of the discourses of childbirth. *Midwifery* 9, 225–34.

Inch, S. and Garforth, S. 1989: Establishing and maintaining breastfeeding. In Chalmers, I., Enkin, M. and Keirce, M.J.N.C. (eds), *Effective care in pregnancy and childbirth*. Oxford: Oxford University Press, 1359–74.

Jacoby, A. 1988: Mother's views about information and advice in pregnancy and childbirth: findings from a national study. *Midwifery* 4, 103–10.

Kirkham, M.J. 1983a: Admission in labour: teaching the patient to be patient? *Midwives Chronicle* February 44–5.

Kirkham, M.J. 1983b: Labouring in the dark: limitations on the giving of information to enable patients to orientate themselves to the likely events and timescale of labour. In Wilson Barnett, J. (ed.), *Nursing research: ten studies in patient care.* Chichester: John Wiley, 81–99.

Kirkham, M. 1989: Midwives and information giving during labour. In Robinson, S. and Thomson, A.M. (eds), *Midwives, research and childbirth*, Vol. 1. London: Chapman and Hall, 117–38.

McKay, S. and Yager Smith, S. 1993: 'What are they talking about? Is something wrong?' Information sharing during the second stage of labour. *Birth* 20(3),142–7.

Rajan, L. 1993: The contribution of professional support, information and consistent correct advice to successful breast feeding. *Midwifery* 9, 197–209.

Stamp, G.E. and Crowther, C.A. 1994: Women's views of their postnatal care by midwives at an Adelaide Women's Hospital. *Midwifery* 10, 148–56.

Further reading

Department of Health 1993: *Report of the Maternity Services Part 2: Survey of good communications practice in maternity services.* London: HMSO.

Hunt, S. and Symonds, A. 1995: *The social meaning of midwifery.* Basingstoke: Macmillan.

9

Assertiveness

Assertiveness is a significant part of communicating for both midwives and those with whom they communicate, particularly women using the maternity services. Health in part depends on being able to consider different ideas; it is about feeling confident in the health decisions that we make, and about being able to make those decisions about how we wish our lives to unfold, and living with the consequences of our actions. It is also a way of dealing with stress in the form of difficult work or family situations.

However, there are broader issues involved in assertiveness. Assertive behaviour is not something which we are all at liberty to achieve, even with training, because equality between individuals, a prerequisite to truly assertive behaviour, has yet to be achieved. Although mutual respect may be missing in any human relationship, problems particularly pertinent in this chapter include those involving men and women, people of different races and the able bodied and disabled. Assertiveness is about finding mutually acceptable solutions in difficult situations, where decision-making may be affected by people's various attitudes, approaches and personalities, or by aspects of the environment, such as politics, social issues and economics.

What is assertiveness?

Assertiveness is a state of mind and behaviour where the person or people concerned are able to listen to and understand what is going on around them, and feel at ease with themselves in their response. Being assertive is about being able to express opinions with confidence, and hear other opinions and opposing views with equanimity. To be assertive it is important to be relatively decisive; although some people will assertively state their right to be confused! So in essence, assertiveness is about finding a balance in life between speaking out and staying quiet, making a decision to act or making a decision to wait; feeling happy and confident with oneself and reasonably popular with others.

Having said all this, it would be a tall order for a person to be assertive all of the time. This is simply unrealistic, as there are all sorts of pressures in life that make all of us react unassertively from time to time – for instance appearing to accept advice that someone offers us when we have no intention of acting on it, or caving in when a colleague makes an unreasonable request of us which it feels easier to carry through than argue about the whys and wherefores. 'An assertive person' for most of us is someone who is generally a good listener, a fairly articulate speaker, and a reasonably confident person. Exercise 9.1 invites reflection about when we are at our most and least assertive, bearing these points in mind.

Nevertheless, it would be difficult for a midwife with very passive or very aggressive tendencies in her communication with others to be an effective health promoter, because of the feelings she would engender in others by her approach. In being passive, she may allow others to make all the important decisions and blame her when things do not go well. Individuals who behave passively in dynamic, important relationships such as those that a midwife has, often find themselves pushed into unpopular jobs or tasks, and may end up feeling upset and resentful without realizing why. On the other hand, a midwife with aggressive tendencies will probably find (although she may not notice) that people generally avoid her, or have arguments with her at regular intervals. In either case, the quality of communication is badly affected, and important messages needlessly lost.

Why is assertiveness important?

Perhaps assertiveness issues have been so popular in midwifery education in recent years because midwives have not felt able to be as assertive, or have as healthily assertive relationships with women and their families as they would wish. But it is not just midwives who have shown interest in assertiveness issues over recent years. Classes especially for women

---

EXERCISE 9.1 When are you at your most and least assertive?

Consider the following points in relationship to yourself.

- What do you do if someone pushes into a queue in front of you?
- How often do you lose your temper with or in front of other people?
- How do you feel when you walk into a room full of people whom you have not previously met?
- How much do you join in in group discussions?
- How do you respond when somebody compliments you?
- Do you feel your best friends understand you well?
- When you meet a stranger, do you tend to introduce yourself, or wait for them to say something?
- If you feel a colleague is being treated unfairly at work, what do you do?
- How do you respond to a colleague who does not pull his/her weight at work?
- How do pushy salespeople make you feel?
- Do you ever make decisions for other people at work?

And perhaps most importantly of all, how would you expect an assertive person to respond in these situations? One of the difficulties of assertive behaviour is measuring it, because there are many assertive responses to any given situation, and assertiveness itself is a very elusive concept, made up of many different human characteristics.

---

have sprung up all over the place, because women seem to feel that they have a particular need to speak out more, and be heard.

Assertiveness is important because if we single it out as a desirable characteristic and consider how a greater degree of assertiveness can be achieved in us as individuals, we are more likely to achieve more assertive relationships with others and our self-esteem and confidence in communicating can only be improved. This will have a knock-on effect in making communication at home and in the workplace more effective, so everyone will be happier – and less frustrated, less disappointed and less discontented.

O'Brien (1990) suggests that assertiveness is useful in the following situations:

- dealing with conflict
- negotiation

- leadership and motivation
- giving and receiving feedback
- cooperative working
- being heard in meetings.

In the arena of health promotion, assertiveness is particularly important because it is a prerequisite for people to change their health behaviour. For instance, having received information about healthier lifestyles in pregnancy, and accepted that a better diet, more exercise, etc. are desirable, a decision must be made enabling that person to modify her behaviour. The confidence and decision-making required to succeed in such a behaviour modification are borne out of assertiveness – a state of feeling in some control of one's life and able to change.

Bond (1991) suggests that as the pace of technological development continues in health care there is going to be a greater need for health professionals such as midwives to be advocates for women. The health care system is going to become more difficult to understand, a greater requirement for informed choice is going to require the midwife to make sure women have access to information which they understand, and women's most simple requests will still need to be taken into consideration. The case for assertive midwives is strong.

The assertive midwife

An assertive midwife is one who respects the integrity of those around her, plays her part in the team effectively, and plays a full part in formulating policy and procedure, where these exist, in her workplace.

However, certain challenges need to be made about how female midwives (the majority in the profession) align their feminine role with that of their professional role, because society still has certain expectations of women, for example to be tender, kind and accommodating, not overambitious, and willing to follow a husband when he gets a new job in a different part of the country regardless of the effect on the woman's own career. Incidentally the sexism which female midwives face has repercussions for male midwives who do not necessarily have an easier time in their professional relationships because of their gender. Indeed, many male midwives find their sexual orientation questioned because they have chosen to pursue a profession with a role defined by society as 'feminine'. They may then be criticized if perceived as being heterosexual – 'What sort of a man are you?' or 'What pleasure do you get from this job?' or criticized if they are perceived as homosexual, as being unmanly, and a threat to society's understanding of the meaning of masculinity. As society appears to accept the male obstetrician much more easily (although not universally), and rarely questions his sexual orientation, a double standard must be operating here – medicine as a caring occupation is acceptable as 'manly', but midwifery is not.

Assertiveness is fundamentally based on the right of each person to function as an equal, and in a less than equal society it is difficult for all but the most confident of women to function outside the boundaries of the social expectations for her sex. (Despite changes in the law on sex discrimination in the 1970s, 25 years later women's average gross weekly pay in full-time employment is still only 72 per cent that of men's pay in Great Britain (Low Pay Unit, 1995). The fact that women are in lower paid jobs than men, and are often paid less than men doing the same or a similar job, is testimony to society's view of women as less than equal in social and financial standing.) Women being asked to make tea or take the minutes at important meetings, entering lower paid caring jobs and professions, being referred to at work as 'a girl' and midwives being expected to clean dirty trolleys left by busy doctors, are all practical manifestations of society's expectations of women.

The importance of assertiveness for midwives also manifests itself in relationships with the users of the maternity services. The ability to hear accurately and acknowledge what is said, treat people as of equal worth, and feel comfortable with people making their own decisions (especially those which run counter to our advice), are all important aspects of an assertive relationship.

However, although it is important for midwives to be aware of the very difficult and complicated equality issues in society which affect everybody's ability to be assertive, that knowledge and awareness can be used positively to build better relationships with both women and colleagues.

The assertive woman

It is difficult for a pregnant woman to be assertive when faced with 'experts' in an unknown environment at a very emotionally vulnerable time. Some of the problems that pregnant women and midwives face are similar – those of society's expectations of women's role and behaviour. But added to this, the childbearing woman may be frustrated by having been kept waiting for an appointment, stripped of her own clothes, or confused by the language she is hearing. It is practically impossible for a woman to meet health professionals on an equal footing unless they demonstrate that they consider her so, but even then for many women it is difficult to express wishes and ideas. Some midwives and other health professionals are trying to improve the situation by providing more information, meeting women and couples in their own home, encouraging the women to wear their own clothes in hospital and using everyday language rather than medical jargon (which, as we have seen in Chapter 9, is more easily said than done).

Unfortunately, when women do speak out confidently about what they want from the maternity services, they are sometimes labelled as 'difficult' or 'aggressive'. The NHS has a historic culture of paternalism or 'doctor/health professional knows best' attitudes and it is only relatively recently that these attitudes have been modified and lay people encouraged to participate more in health care both at a personal and local organizational level. Attitudes and power relationships do not disappear overnight, and assertive behaviour in health service users is sometimes tolerated, but rarely welcomed.

A further limit to the wishes of women being articulated is social class. It is well documented that the higher her social class, the more able the woman is to verbalize her wishes and needs. Women from lower social groups are often treated differently by health professionals too; they are given fewer explanations, fewer choices, and are often subject to stereotyped views about their previous knowledge and intelligence.

Women from ethnic minorities can also find themselves at a disadvantage in an alien maternity service. As well as the possible language barrier, they too may face the prospect of being given fewer explanations and choices. Assertiveness always has a cultural context, and much of the behaviour valued and displayed by Western women is viewed with horror by women from cultures where subservience among women is highly valued. Disabled women may also face particular barriers, such as being given limited information by health professionals who assume intellectual impairment, or paternalistic treatment by those who assume that such women are not capable of protecting their own interests.

It is not always easy for midwives and other health professionals to form relationships based on the respect and personal autonomy necessary for people to assert themselves, however strongly they wish to support a woman in any given situation. Consider the following case which takes place in the delivery suite of a consultant unit:

> Stephanie, a midwife, asks Joanne, who is in labour, if she may perform her next four-hourly routine vaginal examination. Joanne declines, on the basis that observations on both herself and the baby are satisfactory, and she would not consent to any intervention offered at the present time, whatever the result of the examination.

Although many midwives would consider Joanne perfectly within her right and would respect her decision, others may react differently. A host of other issues cloud this situation. If the senior midwife or doctor is critical of the non-active management of labour, or is concerned about relieving labour beds as quickly as possible in the delivery suite to prevent unsafe workloads, Stephanie may find herself in an uncomfortable situation. She may wish to support Joanne but may feel uncomfortable about the reaction she gets when she communicates to other staff the care she has given, who she feels may press her on why she did not make clearer to Joanne the importance of the examination, or the 'dangers' of not knowing Joanne's exact progress. Her own discomfort may lead her to persuade Joanne to have that examination – the price to maintain a quiet life, and avoid a potential confrontation.

This and similar situations are enacted in maternity units on a daily basis throughout the country, and demonstrate the progress needed to make relationships between health carers and recipients more equal. The task, although a daunting one, is being addressed by some health professionals, often through the forum of parent education where assertiveness issues are actively acknowledged and confronted. This acknowledgement will be, for some women, the stimulus they need to consider how they can function more effectively in their dealings with people but should be diplomatically handled so as not to offend women who, for whatever reason, find it impossible to contemplate disagreement.

Building equal relationships

An important part of assertiveness is accepting the equality of each party in any communication, and accepting that everyone has a right to her say, however uncomfortable this is to others. One notable exception to this right to one's say is the attempt to incite inequality in others, for instance by racism, sexism or ageism. O'Brien (1990) suggests the following Bill of Rights:

Everyone has

- the right to be treated with respect
- the right to have and to express her/his own opinions and feelings
- the right to be listened to and taken seriously
- the right to set her/his own priorities
- the right to say 'no' without feeling guilty
- the right to ask for what she/he wants
- the right to ask for information from professionals
- the right to make mistakes
- the right to choose not to assert oneself.

The most important thing about such a list is that the rights are those of everybody, not just the person reading them. Also, with rights come responsibility – responsibility towards ourselves and others, treating others in respectful ways, and indeed as we would wish to be treated ourselves.

However it is difficult to treat people equally in terms of their rights if we do not feel of equal human worth ourselves. The fact that one individual thinks another is more talented, more intelligent, more educated, more wealthy, more assertive, more good-looking, etc. does not make that person of more human worth, and valuing people as of the same worth is important.

Dealing with situations involving people who disagree when consensus is required

Midwives often find themselves in situations where different opinions abound and a single choice of action needs to be agreed. Whether this is for agreement over a new hospital procedure, advocacy in supporting the wishes of a labouring woman or debate over how a health promotion intervention should be initiated, it is important for all parties to be heard even if all their wishes cannot be adopted. All too often in the past midwives have allowed medical and other professional representation to rule the day, but the wishes and attitudes of childbearing women and midwives are receiving greater attention lately. This is because women and midwives are becoming better at stating their needs, and insisting that these are taken seriously and acted upon.

It is only right that the health decisions in maternity care should be taken by people from a variety of backgrounds – all interested professional groups as well as the women who are affected by any decisions. Midwives may find themselves chairing such groups, or feeling a great responsibility within the group in finding shared values, perhaps where at first the separate values seem incompatible. A degree of assertiveness is required both to be heard and to listen to others carefully. Although it is unlikely that everyone will feel happy with the final decision, a group that can manoeuvre itself into a reasonably agreed 'win–win' situation (where at least nobody feels a loser) will have functioned reasonably successfully.

Summary of key points

- Health in part is enhanced by being able to consider different ideas and to make decisions based on the information received. Assertiveness enables us to feel more confident in our relationships and communication with others and is a prerequisite for modifying health behaviour.
- Assertiveness is a state of mind and behaviour where the person or people concerned are able to hear and understand what is going on around them, and feel at ease with themselves in their response.
- To behave assertively necessarily involves the implicit belief that people are all of equal worth, and should be treated with respect. There are deep and fundamental issues involved in maternity care which cannot be easily resolved. The problems of sexism, racism and paternalism militate against the formation of such assertive relationships between women and midwives, women and doctors and midwives and doctors.

- Problems of behaving assertively are compounded for midwives in the difficulties of aligning the professional and feminine role, and for pregnant women in being given limited appointment times with busy professionals in an unfamiliar clinical environment, being subjected to alien language and on occasions being stripped of their normal clothing.
- There are a number of ways in which midwives are addressing assertiveness issues. As well as studying the concept of assertiveness through education and training, they may organize their practice so that they see more women with their families at home, encourage and give women opportunities to express their wishes and needs, provide opportunities to involve interpreters where necessary and use everyday language in their professional conversations. Assertiveness can also be addressed through parent education programmes which not only acknowledge and confront the issues, but encourage women and their partners to set the agenda, deciding what they wish to discuss and which outside speakers they wish to invite and question. Acknowledging and demonstrating that people are of equal worth, and raising assertiveness as an issue in such programmes will also raise women's awareness of how they can most effectively get the best out of their maternity services.
- Women from cultural backgrounds which highly value female subservience must have their beliefs respected and should not be made to feel uncomfortable.

References

Bond, M. 1991: *Assertiveness for midwives*. London: South Bank University.
Low Pay Unit 1995: Quiet growth in poverty. *New Review of the Low Pay Unit* 36, 8–10.
O'Brien, P. 1990: *A guide to assertiveness*. London: The Industrial Society.

Further reading

Butler, P.E. 1992: *Self-assertion for women*. San Francisco: Harper Collins.
Lloyd, S.R. 1988: *How to develop assertiveness*. London: Kogan Page.
Rakos, R. 1991: *Assertive behaviour: theory, research and training*. London: Routledge.
Sharpe, R. 1989: *Assert yourself*. London: Kogan Page.

10

The education component in health promotion

A large part of promoting health by midwives necessarily involves teaching and learning. In this chapter, attention will be given to how learning occurs. Teaching and learning methods will be discussed, tips to make teaching effective will be suggested and techniques addressed. Some general ethical issues of teaching will be raised. Having knowledge and skills as a midwife do not necessarily make a good teacher, or facilitator of learning. Like much of health promotion and midwifery, effective teaching depends on the effective communication skills of the teacher. These skills have been addressed in Chapter 9 and will not be repeated in this chapter, but need to be considered when studying what makes an effective teacher.

How adults learn

Pregnant women and new parents will learn about birth and parenthood from a number of different sources, and in a number of different ways. One of those sources will be midwives, who hold a heavy responsibility to make any educational opportunity they offer as effective as possible. In order to do so an understanding of how adults learn can enhance that effectiveness.

The most important factors in adult learning are strong motivation, participation and activity. The incorporation of all three is required if

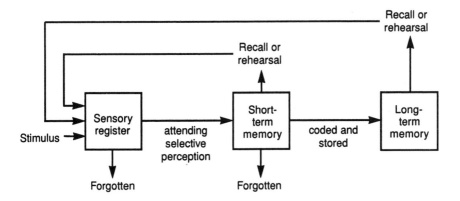

Figure 10.1 An information-processing model of memory (Reproduced from Child, 1993 with kind permission of Cassell)

effective learning is to take place. Motivation to learn about the realities of new parenthood is present in practically all first-time pregnant women and many of their partners as they enter a new phase of their life, and it has little to do with the involvement of a midwife. However if motivation is something that is largely decided before the learner reaches the teacher, participation and active learning are certainly not. A major part of a teacher's responsibility is to enable these to happen in ways that encourage learning by understanding and remembering knowledge and information, by being able to apply it to appropriate situations, and by gaining independence in setting up situations in which participants feel confident to use their new-found knowledge to change their lives for the better.

In order to understand how people learn, it is useful for teachers to understand how they can influence memory retention. Psychologists differentiate between short-term and long-term memory. Child (1993) offers an information-processing model of memory as shown in Fig. 10.1 and describes encoding, storage and retrieval of information in the memory. Encoding is the process by which information is scanned for meaning and relevance, and categorized according to how it will be remembered by associating it with information already stored. For instance, if care of the newborn infant is being discussed, the learner will reflect on her experience of babies and what she has been told by friends and relatives, and store any new information she finds relevant in the same part of her memory. It is hypothesized by psychologists that information will pass through the short-term memory as it is filtered to decide whether it will then be stored in the long-term memory. Factors affecting this differentiation include relevance, interest, good concentration and appeal in the way in which the information is presented, which are likely to result in long-term storage, and lack of interest or relevance, tiredness, pain or overstimulation of the mind which are likely to result in short-term memorizing only.

Retrieval of information occurs when remembered information returns to, or is retrieved from the short-term or working memory, the cue for retrieval being either an external stimulus or a conscious will by the person to search through their memory store for information.

The implications of understanding how memory works for the teacher are that she should ensure as far as possible the comfort of participants, and not overload them with information. It is imperative that participants understand information and see its relevance before they can memorize it, and if they can question, discuss and better still perform an activity associated with the new information, they will memorize its relevant components more effectively.

Learning and storing information for retrieval at a later date is further enhanced by activity such as handling the equipment being explained, or participative discussion of a topic area. As well as helping initially to store the information, actively making use of the information will help it to be retained for longer, and refined to attain greater relevance. It should always be remembered by the teacher that the educational information that a pregnant women stores in her memory has to compete for space with a host of different types of memorized information: childhood memories, telephone messages and shopping lists, social engagements and knowledge of how to perform everyday tasks, not to mention worries about the pregnancy and things she has been told in her antenatal appointments.

Therefore what each woman learns in an antenatal class or in discussion with a midwife early in her pregnancy, could be forgotten later on if she has not retrieved the knowledge and topped it up with new insights, angles or material. For this reason, it helps people to learn if the teacher returns to the same subject at a later date, or in the case of a single session with learners, summarizes important points at the end.

Other factors influencing learning include the pace of the educational encounter, the style of teaching (discussed later in this chapter), the availability of written information to back up verbal interaction, social problems of participants (which may interfere with the learning process), and the intelligence and confidence of the learner in her ability to retain and use information.

Teaching and learning methods

Midwives spend a great deal of their time in one-to-one relationships with women, or with couples. Some of this time will be spent teaching, and there is increasing evidence that one-to-one teaching and information-sharing, tuned into a woman's needs, can be very effective. However, in many situations where it is used it is also necessary because of the personal and private nature of the discussion.

Suitable topics for such individual discussion (and perhaps discussion with a couple seen as a single unit can be included here) include hazards of smoking and strategies for smoking cessation, sexual, family planning and personal issues and infant feeding, where information and advice will need to be tailored to the woman's needs as well as common and research knowledge. All these areas concern attitudes as well as knowledge in influencing behaviour, and these attitudes will need to be acknowledged and incorporated into any information-sharing in order to enhance the effect of decision-making and change, where these are appropriate, in the woman's life.

Realistically much of the midwife's work will involve groups, where there is great advantage to be gained from sharing experiences, views and feelings. Although time constraints will mean that a lot of teaching and learning that may have been better approached with individuals has to occur in groups, the midwife must be able to capitalize on this situation and make the best of it.

There are many ways of giving and sharing information, and the teaching method needs to be suited to the learning requirement in order to be optimally effective. Good teaching usually encompasses a number of approaches, the most common of which are discussed in the following paragraphs.

Discussion

Discussion is a good way to start any teaching and learning activity, whatever the size of the group. It can be used for introducing people to each other and acquainting them with an outline of the session or course content, checking participants' previous levels of knowledge and experience, and sharing attitudes, setting agendas and time limits and the many other aspects of information-sharing.

It is useful for the teacher to have in her mind some trigger questions and topics to keep the discussion flowing. When starting to teach groups, student midwives and midwives are often nervous about discussion 'drying up' and leaving long, awkward silences, or alternatively getting out of hand and moving away from the point. Confidence comes with practice, and once used to feeling comfortable in front of a group, helping interactions and organizing sessions, most teachers find discussion very enjoyable and learn a lot about themselves!

A few of the more difficult situations to cope with during group discussion for the teacher are:

- when one or two people have a lot to say and dominate the proceedings;

- when someone vehemently disagrees with what is said, or gives examples of horror stories;
- when some people do not contribute at all, and worse still look terribly bored, snooze, or break off to talk in smaller, disruptive huddles.

These situations often need to be dealt with speedily and tactfully, so that group cohesion can be maintained and developed. Preventing the situations occurring by agreeing ground rules at the beginning and reminding participants of them as the session progresses is useful, as are general questions such as 'Would anyone else like to comment on that?', or 'Is it useful to you all to proceed with this line of discussion?'.

Group work

One of the main problems with discussion in larger groups is that some members will be too shy or retiring to contribute, and it will be impossible for the teacher to know whether they are receiving any benefit from the session unless she singles them out, which they may find acutely embarrassing. Group work is a good way to make sure that everyone takes part by organizing participants to work together in groups of two to four. The shy ones can then discuss the topic without having to expose their nervousness or ideas to everyone all at once. Again, planning is of the essence – groups need to be clear about what their objectives are, as the teacher cannot maintain a constant presence in each group. Groups can be asked to report back to the larger group through an elected spokesperson or may keep the details of their group discussion to themselves. It is important to agree and set a time limit on group activities to give an idea of depth of discussion required in order to reduce the risk of irrelevant discussion, although some would argue that any discussion which the small group members choose to have in the allotted time is, by the fact of its having occurred, useful to them.

Role-play

Role-play is a learning activity that most adults either love or hate. It is undoubtedly effective in helping people to understand both their own and other people's feelings and emotions in areas such as job interviews, assertiveness and breaking bad news, but can feel very threatening to shy or private individuals.

It makes learning very active and when tactfully introduced and prepared for, participants may be pleasantly surprised at the advantages it has to offer, in terms of universal participation, developing confidence in working out practical solutions to otherwise apparently insoluble problems, and sharing and demonstrating problem-solving approaches to both personal and professional dilemmas. As well as in health education, role-play is becoming more widely incorporated into nurse and midwife education, for instance in learning about antenatal booking interview skills, assertiveness training and preceptor/assessor training skills. It can be used in antenatal groups, for instance in couples self-counselling and assertiveness training, but needs to be introduced and controlled with great diplomacy as, if participants feel uncomfortable with it, they are unlikely to turn up for the rest of the classes. It may be beneficial for two teachers, or a teacher and a volunteer learner, to role-play a situation for discussion by the whole group, and this can lead to humorous as well as educational follow-on discussions.

Role-play is not suitable for groups where trust among members is yet to be built, or very large groups where the backgrounds of the individuals are not known and role-play introduced in any form, may cause great personal upset.

Lecture

The lecture as a teaching strategy has become less popular in recent years because its didactic approach does not allow for contemporaneous inter-action or debate. It is the teaching method least suited to adult needs because it involves no participation on the part of the learner who has no influence on the pace of its delivery, and whilst proceeding takes no account of learner progress or the need for activity to maintain concentra-tion and aid understanding and memory retention. However it can be used very effectively where a lecturer is particularly knowledgeable, or as the least of all evils in a subject suited to such a style such as putting across information, and also to large audiences wishing for relatively simple information, such as couples newly pregnant wishing to gain gen-eral information on local maternity services, where time and numbers constrain the use of a more interactive style of learning.

The lecture allows for greater amounts of information to be put across to large groups, by an 'expert', or a person with in-depth specialist knowledge. A question time at the end can allow for some interaction with the more outgoing members of the audience, but shyer members with pressing questions will be at a disadvantage here.

One of the problems of the lecture is that information given may sound very impressive but may actually be untrue, based on false premises or purely on the opinion of the speaker who, to make her point more forceful, presents it as fact. 'Expertise' itself has become a contentious issue in contemporary society because truth and knowledge are often subjective, culture-based, and movable objects depending on one's own values and beliefs.

Making teaching effective

What makes a teacher or a learning experience exciting, fascinating or inspirational? No doubt our own interest in a subject is crucial to our concentration but some teachers have an almost mesmerizing style, and give the impression of being able to make any subject fascinating. In any teaching situation there are many strategies which all teachers can use consistently to make sessions run more smoothly, and make the learning process more effective for the participants.

Preparation

It is always useful to prepare for any session, not only by updating knowledge, getting visual aids ready and writing prompt notes, but checking the room, that any equipment needed works beforehand and even that the date and time are convenient to the participants. There is nothing more frustrating to learners, or to the teacher, than an overhead projector with a broken bulb, or a chalkboard with no chalk. If the teaching method depended on such equipment being available in good working order, the frustration can continue even after the problem has been solved, putting the teacher off her stride. However, it is possible to be overprepared, by attempting to pre-empt any discussion or debate and by being too strict in following an inflexible plan, when participants feel a strong need to discuss a point which the teacher is only prepared to gloss over quickly. Overpreparation can make a session feel very stilted, although it can feel safer for the teacher.

Preparation also includes having some knowledge of how people learn, and how groups interact. All this information is used to decide on appropriate information to be conveyed and shared, teaching methods and audience involvement. Preparation of the actual material to be conveyed should start with setting objectives, or proposed learning outcomes. Although it is easy to launch in with information about, say, infant feeding, the information may be difficult for the audience to decipher if it is not specific to their needs. For instance, the midwife may spend a lot of time talking about why women choose to breastfeed, when in fact the women have already decided whether to and why – they are more likely to wish to know how to prepare themselves, how to manage breast- or bottle-feeding in the first few days and weeks, how to suppress their milk supply, what early problems they may face, and what resources they have available to deal with any problems. An example of the objectives a midwife may set herself for such a session is given in Table 10.1. Such preparation will not only help the midwife to keep her input relevant, but will also help her to evaluate the success of the session by giving her measurable outcomes.

Table 10.1 Session on infant feeding – learning objectives

At the end of this parent education session on infant feeding, the participants will:

(a) Have a clear understanding of the physiology of breastfeeding, and the production and suppression of the milk supply.
(b) Be clearer in their decision about whether to breast- or bottle-feed, having heard the advantages and disadvantages of both methods of infant feeding.
(c) Gained confidence in their ability to nurture their infant in the way they have chosen.
(d) Be aware of the practical and safety issues in preparing infant formula.
(e) Have had the opportunity to ask any questions about infant feeding in the first few weeks of the baby's life.
(f) Be aware of support people and systems available to them in the first few weeks of parenthood and know how to access that help.

Organization of the material

It is important for learners in most situations to have some structure in the way information is presented, in order to enhance memory retention. Haphazard structure gives learners an extra mental job to do – that of sorting information – which may interfere with memory retention or may even mean missing important information while the mind tries to make order of the previous piece of information. A further useful ground rule for the teacher is to let the participants know the proposed structure at the beginning of the session, or agree one with them, so they can more easily and confidently follow the teacher's line of thinking. Obviously the teacher should then try to stick to this agenda, and keep discussion and information-sharing relevant.

Important points should be made early in the session when concentration is at its highest. Key points can be stressed by voice inflection, writing them down for participants to see, or giving them out on a handout. The temptation to give too much information should be avoided, especially when the group is looking at an area of new information. Medical and health jargon should also be avoided.

Paying attention to the needs of the group

An effective teacher will be aware that the group is not a static, accepting entity. Feelings of individuals within the group to and for each other will be changing and changeable. Learning may be enhanced or interfered with by group dynamics, some of which will be conscious, and some subconscious. Teachers may have some influence over tolerance levels and opinions within the group by the inevitable exposure of their own feelings and attitudes. Although in optional adult education, such as parent education, participants will on the whole take responsibility for their own relationships and learning within the group, it is useful for teachers to assess their own responsibility, if any, in enhancing group cohesion.

Members of the group will learn in different ways and at different paces, so using different teaching styles will not only add variety to the teaching, but provide a wider range of appeal to the group.

Paying attention to individuals

Individual needs within a group can be very various and one of the more sensitive skills of a teacher can be to develop not only knowledge, but confidence and decision-making skills in each individual, by using strategies to involve everyone at some level in the learning process. By using a variety of teaching methods, as well as eye contact and voice to embrace the whole group and maintain concentration, discussion, handing round models, asking opinions and many other ploys can help participants to feel an important and integral part of the group.

It is also important to be aware of the comfort of all the participants. Although a nervous teacher may feel preoccupied with her own performance, awareness and verbal acknowledgement of the comfort of others will enable them to feel more comfortable and better able to concentrate. Starting a session with 'Let me know, anyone, if the room gets too hot so we can open a window' or 'These chairs are very hard – shall we break for coffee early so no one gets too uncomfortable?' will do much to put people at ease, and perhaps this move towards informality will also help the teacher to relax. Observing concentration rates will also enable the teacher to assess her interest rating with participants and to have breaks or a change in teaching method at appropriate times.

Making learning fun

There is no reason why learning shouldn't be enjoyable. For some people it may be their first experience of formal learning since school, and they may not have very high expectations of really enjoying themselves. However, it is always worth considering how sessions can be made fun, as this will enhance learning and the participants' return to any future similar sessions. Although not every midwife who teaches health promotion will feel able personally to keep her audience amused for great lengths of time, midwives generally have many fascinating anecdotal stories to tell (perhaps adding a few details by artistic licence to make the story a little more interesting and protect confidentiality) about her practice. However, it is vital that confidences are protected when case histories are given, and worth bearing in mind that nobody wants to feel they might be the next person as the subject of a midwife's tale!

The use of humour can also take on a broader role. Light-hearted banter often occurs in general conversation and, as well as breaking up chunks of factual information, helps people to relax and learn about each other. The humorous atmosphere does not necessarily need to come from the teacher – although her demeanour will have some influence on the seriousness or otherwise of the occasion: participants' comments may lighten the situation.

When using posters, overhead projections or slides, cartoons can be amusing and aid learning and memory.

Enthusiasm and the teacher

Learners evaluate teacher enthusiasm very highly – very often it is top of the list when learners are asked to rank order their preferred teacher attributes. It can make a dull subject interesting, and the teacher worth listening to. Perceived lack of enthusiasm may be misconstrued as lack of interest in the subject, and the learners too may lose their enthusiasm to learn.

Evaluating each session

Without assessing one's teaching it is impossible to know what was done well, and what could be improved on. Evaluation can be formal or informal, done by the teacher on herself or by asking the participants, or by an outside agency. All have their advantages and disadvantages.

Simply asking participants how the session has gone for them and giving them time to respond is quick but may not elicit criticism and ideas for improvement, especially if they do not feel it is a safe enough environment. (Knowing the midwife whose teaching they are critical of may care for them in labour the following week will be much too uncomfortable for some people.) Written evaluations may be more revealing, but take longer to design (unless invited on a blank sheet of paper), complete and analyse. Anonymity may lead to a better response, but comments must then remain confidential, and unreturned forms cannot be retrieved.

Self-evaluation by the teacher is always useful if honestly considered, in reflecting on how a particular course or session went. Some self-directed questions are suggested in Table 10.2. Self-evaluation should also reflect whether the objectives set in the planning stage have been fully or partially met.

All evaluations, however formulated, should be followed up by an action plan of practical ways to improve future teaching. Evaluation therefore becomes cyclical.

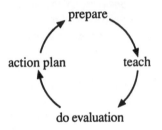

Table 10.2 Self-evaluation of a teaching session

What things did I do particularly well?
 – Why did they go well?

Which parts of the session didn't go so well?
 – Why didn't they go well?
 – How could I improve them in future sessions?

How did the discussion flow?

What was my body language?
What did the body language of the participants convey to me?

What teaching/learning style(s) evoked the most lively response from the participants?

Did I allow for the needs of individuals/the group to be expressed, and answered?

With the benefit of hindsight, were the teaching aids used appropriate? Could they be improved, or changed for something more suitable?

Did any fathers present, look comfortable/uncomfortable?

The use of visual aids in teaching and learning

Visual and other teaching aids invariably enhance the quality of the learning experience by broadening the learners' sensory input from merely looking and listening to seeing, touching and even smelling and tasting. Generally speaking, the simpler the aid is the better, as more people will understand its concept and the point it is making will be clearer. Aids that can be handed around, handled or used to help people experience a situation before they find themselves in it 'for real', such as breathing into an Entonox mask before labour, both concentrate attention and allow for questions to be raised at an early stage in the development of knowledge.

Common visual aids such as posters, slides, chalkboards, videos and leaflets are almost always appreciated by the audience to view and read at leisure. Touchable aids such as a doll and pelvis, cervical dilation chart and aromatherapy oils have also been traditionally popular in antenatal and midwifery education, but audiences and participants often particularly enjoy the very individual aids that some teachers design themselves and employ in their teaching, for instance a one-woman role-play, a homemade doll or uterus, or a simple household item used to demonstrate physiological or anatomical detail.

Priest and Schott (1991) suggest that the best visual aid for parent educators is our own body. Examples of using ourselves as illustrations include:

- showing where the diaphragm, coccyx, symphysis pubis and pelvic brim are and then encouraging participants to find their own;
- showing the length and location of a Caesarean scar with a neat, small gesture on our own body;
- holding a doll up against our own body to show lie and engagement;
- demonstrating exercises, for instance to help backache.

Teaching practical skills

Midwives are very often involved in teaching practical skills to pregnant women and new mothers and fathers, such as urine-testing, breast- and bottlefeeding and sterilizing equipment for the new baby, and babycare. Knowledge of how practical skills are best taught and learnt will enhance the effectiveness of such a session. Ewles and Simnett (1995) described three stages, demonstration by the teacher, rehearsal by the learner(s) and practice by the learner(s), as the most effective in aiding such learning.

If a group can be small enough that everyone can have a go at the task immediately, memory of its performance will be enhanced; if not, demonstration by the teacher is highly recommended in some visual form. A description by the teacher of a practical task, with no teaching aids, is not likely to be remembered and at worse, vital steps in the process may be forgotten. As the Chinese proverb goes:

I hear and I forget,
I see and I remember,
I do and I understand.

ssues in health education

o one would disagree that teaching and learning are important human development, as in all areas of health promotion there l issues involved, awareness of which may provoke a deeper leve... understanding of processes and problem-solving, and therefore the quality of the teaching and learning process.

One ethical dimension of education which increases awareness of a wider world is that the new horizons can lead to increased expectations, and many parentcraft programmes are criticized for giving an idealized view of birth, which can in reality be a painful, frustrating and disappointing process. A particular problem may be encouraging participants to be assertive and questioning when in practice their stance may not be respected, and their questions may remain unanswered, leading to disappointment that could be avoided if expectations had not been raised in the first place. However, radical education theory questions the traditional role of the teacher as a controller of information and knowledge and favours the 'teacher' being a facilitator of learning, whose responsibility is to provide a psychological climate in which the learner is able to take personal control of her learning, and any repercussions from it. The experience or process of learning becomes something more than a static goal, and the learner questions at her own pace, and evaluates the answers she gets in her own way.

The teacher has some responsibility in how she fields the questions of her audience. For instance, her body language and replies may encourage non-threatening questioning and discourage assertive or difficult questions. In Chapter 9, Mavis Kirkham's research on communication by midwives working in the delivery suite was discussed, and examples given of how midwives respond to questions. One conversation she describes (1989) goes as follows:

Woman: Is there only one sort of injection?
Midwife: Don't be thinking six hours or four hours ahead. See how it goes.
          I say see how it goes. (Changes subject.)

This example can be used to demonstrate how the deflection of a request for information may inhibit a woman asking for further information. The frustration the woman felt in the response she received can only be imagined, but good preparation for childbirth, including an understanding of the role of her allocated midwife during labour, may have given her the confidence to rephrase the question and press for a more adequate response. Although it may seem idealistic, there are ethical responsibilities involved for all midwives in their teaching role to facilitate learning, as well as provide and share information. The real meanings of facilitation, relinquishing control and giving power to learners (together with their right to disagree and make mistakes) can only take on importance to the new teacher over time, with experience and with deep thought.

An ethical issue on the subject of parent education programmes that has concerned midwives for some time, is the underrepresentation of the lower socio-economic groups. McIntosh (1988) has suggested that this is because the classes are not perceived as valuable, and although various solutions have been put forward, such as classes being held in community centres rather than hospitals, one-to-one teaching in the home and providing crèches during classes, initiatives have been largely unsuccessful in balancing social groups by achieving higher attendance in women from backgrounds of traditionally low participation, except in places like Cowgate, Newcastle (*see* Chapter 3), where social disadvantage is strongly acknowledged in the group and the midwives perform some social work, as well as midwifery work.

Women whose first language is not English and teenagers are also underrepresented in parent education groups, as well as in antenatal clinics in early pregnancy. Valuable educational opportunities are therefore often lost. Again, midwives can do much to improve facilities for such women, many of whom do wish to attend some sort of group with people with whom they feel comfortable. Teenage pregnancy groups which encourage discussion (rather than teacher controlled 'lectures' which young people may be keen to avoid), and groups with link workers present to interpret for women who do not speak English can do much to inform women who may otherwise not gain such benefits from the health services.

Summary of key points

- A significant part of the midwife's role involves information-sharing and raising awareness of health issues. Some of this is done informally, and much occurs formally in parent education sessions.
- A good teacher is one who facilitates learning. This skill is mainly dependent on the effective communication of the teacher and her ability to see herself as a resource in the learning process rather than a gatekeeper of information.
- The most important factors in adult learning are motivation, participation and activity. While motivation in a learner is largely predetermined, participation and activity are dependent in formal teaching on the way the teacher facilitates the session.
- When people hear new information, their brain will scan the message for relevance and store a memory only if the information is personally

interesting and meaningful. The memory can be retrieved at a later date when it is triggered by an external stimulus or conscious will.

- Blocks to learning and remembering information include lack of interest or relevance, tiredness, pain, overstimulation of the mind, the pace being too fast or too slow, non-participatory information-giving, and lack of confidence by the participant in her ability to retain and use the information.

- Where a midwife is involved in leading formal learning groups such as parent education sessions, she has a number of teaching and learning methods at her disposal. These include discussion, group work, role-play and lecturing. Each have advantages and disadvantages.

- There are a number of ways in which a midwife may maximize the learning that occurs in groups. She should adequately prepare herself, the participants and the environment. Her material should be organized in a way that demonstrates her understanding of learning processes. As well as paying attention to the needs of the group, she should be sensitive to individuals. Her own enthusiasm will be vital in maintaining participants' interest.

- It is always helpful for the midwife to evaluate her teaching, or facilitating role, to examine what she has done well, and where she can improve.

- Giving learning a visual component increases interest in the subject areas. Visual aids may include a one-woman role-play, a homemade doll and pelvis, or a poster or slide.

- There are a number of ethical issues involved in health education. These include the problems which may be caused in increasing expectations, the way a teacher or facilitator deals with difficult questions and the dilemmas of education not reaching those who may most benefit from increased knowledge and the advantages of group support inherent in group-learning.

References

Child, D. 1993: *Psychology and the teacher*. London: Cassell.

Ewles, L. and Simnett, I. 1995: *Promoting health: a practical guide*. London: Scutari Press.

Kirkham, M. 1989: Midwives and information-giving during labour. In Robinson, S. and Thomson, A.M. (eds), *Midwives, research and childbirth*, Vol. 1. London: Chapman and Hall, 117–38.

McIntosh, J. 1988: A consumer view of birth preparation classes. *Midwives Chronicle*, January, 8–9.

Priest, J. and Schott, J. 1991: *Leading antenatal classes*. Oxford: Butterworth-Heinemann.

Further reading

Combes, G. and Schonveld, A. 1992: *Life will never be the same again: a review of antenatal and postnatal health education*. London: Health Education Authority.
Wilson, P. 1990: *Antenatal teaching. A guide to theory and practice*. London: Faber and Faber.

Part III

Transforming health promotion theory into midwifery practice

Introduction

There follow five chapters by midwives and health professionals with a special interest in the health of childbearing women, and the promotion of health in practice.

In the opening chapter Patricia Wilson explores with a number of women their attitudes to the health advice which they received during pregnancy. In this small study the interviews raise some interesting issues for midwives in considering to what depth we should find out about each woman's circumstances and lifestyle, the nature of the support that women want and how we can best serve each woman in our care when resources may be very stretched. Midwives must often wonder, after they have completed an antenatal booking or postnatal visit, packed with their own health advice, what women actually do with the information they have been exposed to. This chapter delves under the surface of what these women actually reflected on in the weeks following consultations with professionals, and in turn may help health professionals to consider the most effective ways and times for dispensing health advice. Such advice seems to come in a number of different forms from many sources, and midwives have a responsibility to help women access the information they want and make sense of a plethora of new knowledge which at times can seem contradictory and overwhelming.

Val Thomas next explores current issues in smoking and pregnancy and the role of midwives in helping women to stop smoking. This very practical, evidence-based chapter illustrates how a sound knowledge of the theory behind health promotion can help the midwife to become more effective, and thereby more confident. Importantly, it helps the midwife to differentiate between women who are ready to consider stopping smoking and those who are not, so she can give the right kind of support to each woman.

Maggie McNab tackles the area of sexual health promotion; sexuality, HIV and AIDS, and family planning. An area until recently poorly researched and written about by midwives, sexual health must be considered a major area of interest for those of us concerned with the broad issues of health and its promotion in the childbearing population.

In Chapter 14, Lea Jamieson and Louise Long describe their development of breastfeeding workshops, designed to enhance the knowledge, confidence and skills of mothers and midwives together. Their evaluation of their work adds weight to the need for much greater promotion of breastfeeding, and this project is an innovative way of achieving such promotion.

Finally, Margaret Adams reviews the literature surrounding the causes and predisposing factors to mental ill-health and considers how mental health and well-being can best be promoted in pregnancy and early motherhood, giving examples of best practice in this area of midwifery.

11

Pregnant women's attitudes to health advice

Patricia Wilson

In terms of health promotion, the antenatal period would seem to offer a unique opportunity. Concern for the fetus and the future family are both expressed and implicit in the way women behave during pregnancy and it may be supposed that pregnant women are receptive to health education. As each individual is unique, so will be her response to her pregnancy and it can be observed that not everyone maximizes their chances of a healthy family. To work effectively, health promoters need not only their own knowledge and expertise, but an understanding of what women believe and how they think about health issues. Health in pregnancy cannot be isolated from health in general and some of the research described in this chapter reflects this. It will look at what research has to say about lay perspectives of health, and will also describe the results of a small qualitative study of pregnant women into their feelings about health and health promotion in relation to childbearing.

Lay definitions of and attitudes to health

In health promotion, as in any educative process, the starting point is crucial. John Holt (1984), teacher and educational consultant, illustrated this vividly when he described his experience of helping a child who, in 6 years of school, had made no progress in maths. It was not until he determined the low level of her insight into numbers that she was able to begin to build up her knowledge. This may seem to be far removed from advice to pregnant women, but Holt's comment that this child learned so little because 'no one ever began where she *was*' does have relevance to health promotion.

To try to understand where women are, in terms of beliefs and previous knowledge and experience, we could with profit ask ourselves four questions:

1. How do individuals define health?
2. Do people believe they have power over their own health status?
3. Do they believe they have a responsibility to maintain their own health?
4. Do they wish to pursue health?

How individuals view health and illness will affect their resistance or openness to health promotion. Health is seen in relative, not absolute terms. Health and ill-health are defined socially as well as medically and depend on individual or family circumstances. Definitions usually contain some positive elements, however the negative element is always represented in some form of absence of disease (Herzlich, 1973; Pill and Stott, 1982). The second most common element of lay definitions of health is ability to function, and there can be a division between normal daily functioning and the superior sport fitness (Eadie, 1987). Emotional well-being is included in lay definitions. There is also a moral aspect to health: it is desirable and even where some degree of sickness is present its significance may be minimized (Blaxter and Paterson, 1982), showing a reluctance to accept the sick role and possibly fear of social sanctions (Williams, 1983). Health may also equal happiness, and misery may be seen as an indulgence (Pill and Stott, 1982).

A sense of power over one's health is related partly to beliefs of disease causation and also to a sense of control over life generally. Calnan (1987) asked a mixed-sex, wide-variety group about their beliefs on the causes of specific diseases. The medical model of biological causation of disease predominated and where medical science can provide no clear cause, for example cancer, there was a greater sense of helplessness and fear. Where medicine presented a number of factors causing disease, for example heart disease, although there was recognition of the possibility of control through factors such as smoking, external factors such as genetics, environment and infection predominated and so the degree of control was not perceived to be great. Pill and Stott (1982) identified 'multi-factorial disease causation' but the 'germ theory' was predominant and, on balance, there were more causes thought by individuals to be outside their control. Some factors, for example poor eating habits leading to increased vulnerability to illness, were seen to be within an individual's control, but many people felt vulnerability to disease had more to do with genetics or a person's given constitution.

Each person, through upbringing, circumstances and education, will form beliefs about her ability to control her own life and this will influence health behaviour. Allison (1991) reviews the studies which have used theoretical models to interpret health behaviour. While he acknowledges the importance of a sense of control he draws attention to the limits of individual control and the dangers of inappropriate expectations.

Taking responsibility for health is linked to beliefs about health. It is not realistic to accept responsibility if one believes the cause of ill-health to be an external force beyond one's control. In some circumstances responsibility may be admitted, lip service paid to preventive health behaviour but no action is taken.

Calnan (1987) and Pill and Stott (1982) both found that individual responsibility in lifestyle contribution to health was acknowledged and both studies showed a socio-economic class difference. People described by these researchers as 'middle class' were more ready to accept responsibility for neglect, which they saw as increasing vulnerability to disease, but were reluctant to accept that lifestyle was completely within individual control. Those described as 'working class' were more likely to be fatalists who accepted less responsibility for ill-health, with the exception of short-term direct risk-taking. Calnan (1987) found 'ambivalence and contradiction and no coherent theory' about responsibility for health.

Health is important to individuals but rarely a goal in itself. Though desirable, it may not be actively sought if the means to health are not perceived to be within individual control. There is no doubt that absence of disease is seen as desirable, but those individuals who have little belief in their ability to control their lives may disregard illnesses perceived as minor rather than actively seek to improve their health (Blaxter and Paterson, 1982). Those individuals who do seek actively to improve their health through diet and exercise may be seen by others as fanatics. There is some evidence of a balancing of risks and benefits, for example, smoking and lung cancer, where the pleasure and social benefits may be seen as outweighing the risks. However, there may be an element of denial in playing down the perceived risks in the interests of peace of mind, allowing the individual to continue to engage in the chosen behaviour (Calnan, 1987). Health may be regarded as desirable and an essential precondition for a full life, but health-enhancing behaviour will often be ignored if it conflicts with the main life priority of pleasure and enjoyment (Eadie, 1987). For those with an addiction problem the maintenance of the habit and the very short-term benefits so gained are likely to take precedence over any issue of health. Long-term health benefits in the future are often disregarded.

Health as a goal in itself is seen as desirable by few and can be interpreted by others as displaying an unhealthy attitude. Health is desirable in so far as it allows one to function as required by one's circumstances and also allows one to enjoy life.

The interviews

Pregnancy is a time when concern for the well-being of the unborn child is likely to increase susceptibility to health messages. This study, in which eight women were interviewed, was aimed at deepening understanding of the women's perceptions of health messages from whatever source. The intention was to discover what the women perceived these sources to be and which of these sources they rated most highly. Some estimate of the quality and quantity of that advice was also sought.

Table 11.1 Details of the women interviewed

Name	Age	Marital status	Occupation
Diane	38	Married	Pensions administrator
Angela	31	Married	Security officer
Sonia	36	Married	Television director
Elise	32	Married	Personnel manager
Tina	28	Married	Nanny
Jean	27	Unmarried, lives with partner	Graphic designer
Rosie	27	Married but separated	Betting shop assistant
Christine	24	Unmarried, no longer lives with partner	Computer software administrator

The women interviewed (Table 11.1) were recruited on a casual basis (convenience sample) from an antenatal clinic and the study was conducted by means of semi-structured, tape-recorded individual interviews. Their names have been changed to protect identities. The women were all having first babies and when interviewed were more than 28 weeks pregnant. None had any serious medical problems and all gave birth without major complications to healthy babies after the interviews. All spoke fluent English and there was a range of educational standards and work experience. The issues raised were analysed under the themes of stated or implied attitudes to health, attitudes to pregnancy and making changes, relationships with professionals and attitudes to media advice.

The results

Attitudes to health

The women were asked, 'Do you think of yourself as a very health conscious person?' The respondents' estimates of the degree of health consciousness they felt they had matched well with what they said about their health behaviour. All mentioned diet and exercise as health issues. Four raised the issue of smoking and five the drinking of alcohol. Some felt they had become more health conscious since becoming pregnant.

Influence of family from childhood onward was present. Factors seen as negative could act as warnings and result in the women adopting healthier behaviour. Angela recalled that both her parents had heart trouble. 'I was about 14 when their health started deteriorating and advice that was given to them, it's stuck in my mind.' It was acknowledged that within the family situation there is some lack of control by individuals. As Diane said, 'You didn't have a say in what you had to eat, but I didn't always want what I was given'. School was not remembered as having any part in health education. Although exercise was linked to health, school sport was not described by any of the women as a health activity. Partners of this group were not perceived as an influence and the women were more likely to try to influence them.

The development of health behaviour took place in a social context, with observations of and discussions with friends and colleagues playing a part. One woman who commented about drinking implied that possible social censure was significant. Pleasure was an important factor. Enjoyment and the sociable aspects of exercise featured often in the women's comments. The balance between the value put on pleasure and health benefits varied. Elise said, 'If I really didn't like it I wouldn't do it, and yet I'm conscious that I want to keep myself fit'. And Jean reported that she exercised 'Primarily for pleasure. I'm not really one for sport'. When the pleasure or the sociable aspects were diminished this was likely to prevent the activity.

Only one person talked about long-term health. Sonia, who had done aerobics for 10 years said: 'I don't want osteoporosis and all those sort of things when I'm older'.

No direct questions were asked of the women about responsibility for health, but many of the comments about diet, exercise, smoking and alcohol consumption implied some personal responsibility. Some direct comments were made. For example, Sonia said 'You are the governor of your own system and it's absolutely ridiculous to expect the hospital to pick up the pieces'. There was one example of health defined as fitness, coupled with the belief that this fitness may not prevent all illness. Sonia considered that 'some people do get ill, irrespective of health, there are genetic things etc.'. She was also prepared to quantify individual responsibility. 'In my view, three-quarters of your unpleasant health is down to the way you behave.'

No woman saw health as a goal in itself and several implied less than full-hearted approval for those who followed extreme habits in diet or exercise. For example, Jean stated that 'I don't go out of my way to be a "health junkie"'. One woman – Elise – stated her disapproval of obsessive behaviour, but from her opinions and statements about her lifestyle she appeared to be one of the most health conscious of the respondents. She also appeared to hold a balanced view of health maintenance and was the only one who included a mental aspect. She said 'I'm aware of doing the right thing, but not to the point where you push yourself or you deny yourself anything. Mental and emotional well-being are important to health as well, so to seek advice and guidance on those sort of issues may be necessary.'

Attitude to pregnancy and making changes

Most of the respondents were happy to be pregnant, with five having planned, or implied that they had planned to start a family. Two displayed some ambivalent feelings, but appeared at the time of interview to be looking forward to the baby. All the women had made some changes in their health behaviour during the pregnancy. It was either implied or stated that the changes were at least in part for the benefit of the baby. Influences which contributed to the changes could be physiologically changed appetites or preferences, intrinsic feelings or extrinsic pressures.

The three women who had waited longest before starting a family were those who were the most expressive of their feelings. Diane said 'I envisaged if ever I did get pregnant, my pregnancy would be like the icing on the cake, we know that it's a little girl, all my dreams coming true, I just can't wait to meet her'. This contrasts with Elise, who was able to put her plans into action more easily. Her words alone could be interpreted as calculating, but her manner was warm and one of quiet happiness. 'My husband and I have been married for six years and decided now that the time was right, and I looked into preconception care a little beforehand. Career-wise it feels right to take a little break as well.' Two women were no longer with their partners. Rosie had ended an unsatisfactory relationship and Christine had left a violent one. Both women had experienced some ambivalent feelings about the pregnancy, but being pregnant in difficult circumstances did not seem to prevent them from being positive about their babies.

Becoming pregnant was seen by some of the women as an achievement which merited a reward. Diane saw the baby as a sort of bonus in her life which allowed her to indulge in chocolate and ice-cream. 'That's not being very health conscious, but I think I deserve my treats because I'm pregnant.' Difficulties in conceiving did not appear to motivate either Sonia or Angela to adopt healthier lifestyles beforehand. Angela consciously made changes after the pregnancy was confirmed. Sonia commented about making changes in lifestyle and was somewhat self-critical because she had not done all that she felt she could have done.

Three women talked of taking responsibility for the baby as someone who was unable to do so for him/herself and that sense of responsibility was present in all of the women. Elise was probably the most health-conscious both vocally and in her behaviour and also the most relaxed in her approach to that responsibility, but she did imply avoidance of guilt. 'It seems to me that the baby is an incredible parasite and it will keep going, almost regardless of what you do, but I think you always feel better psychologically if you are doing the right things'. Diane was more explicit: 'If there's anything that's my responsibility, it's to make sure that when she's born she's as perfect as she possibly can be. Because I would never ever forgive myself if something happened and it was tracked back to me.' Anxiety and possible guilt about an adverse outcome to pregnancy was sometimes present. Anxiety may remain even when health behaviour changes have been made, due to a lingering fear that the changes may be inadequate or too late, and there was some attempt to rationalize such fears.

Health behaviour changes made after the beginning of pregnancy may be initiated because of physical changes altering appetites or feelings but then continued for health reasons. Christine said 'Smoking left a horrible taste in my mouth then I thought, you're pregnant, you mustn't smoke any more'. Individuals varied in how easy or difficult they found it to make lifestyle changes in pregnancy. Diane, happy in a stable relationship, was confident in her ability to make decisions. Christine, although supported by a caring mother, had broken off a violent partnership and seemed less confident in making decisions and keeping to her good intentions of being healthy. There was little evidence of partners playing much part in the process of making changes. Friends and colleagues had some influence and two women commented that they had responded positively to pressure from people within their social group. However the pressure for 4 years to stop smoking had only worked for Christine after she became pregnant. The influence of others was not always positive and pressure could be resented. Rosie said 'It's my health, if they just left me alone, I'd do it by myself'. Partners, where present, were protective and often anxious for the welfare of mother or baby or both. The women seemed to appreciate this concern. Where partners were not present the woman's mother was the most significant person and fulfilled a similar role.

To breastfeed or not is a health behaviour decision which may be taken in pregnancy. Feelings about breastfeeding could be very strong before pregnancy and remain so but they could also change radically. Reasons for changing views seemed to be intrinsic rather than any educational influence and some of the women were still uncertain. Diane's dramatic reversal of feelings about this issue appeared to be linked to protective and emotional feelings about her baby. Before pregnancy, in spite of knowing about the health benefits of breastfeeding, her feelings were negative. 'Before I got pregnant I thought it was probably one of the most disgusting, horrendous things that anybody could do.' But later, 'I just feel that it's more participation with your baby's growth, the only thing you can do as a mother that nobody else can do and a lovely close bonding'. For Angela, breastfeeding did not appeal, in spite of expecting her very precious, much wanted baby. She argued around her decision to bottle-feed, citing her partner's desire to participate and her plan to return to work early. She stated firm beliefs contrary to current professional advice about the benefits of breastfeeding: 'The latest information that seems to be coming out is, it's just as good with all the different formulas'. But she acknowledged a blocking out of information about breastfeeding.

Most of the respondents intended to breastfeed, knowing about health benefits and wanting to do the best for the baby, although their knowledge was not necessarily extensive. Several wanted to hedge their bets, being aware that problems in initiating breastfeeding do occur. Elise spoke of breastfeeding being a benefit to her health as well as for the baby, believing breastfeeding would assist her to regain her figure more quickly after the birth.

Relationships with professionals

Health professionals were seen as important and reliable sources of information and advice during pregnancy. The women tended to use professionals when they felt the need, but they were not the only sources of advice nor were they necessarily seen as infallible. The women did not seem to expect professionals to meet health advice needs by individual assessment. Of the professionals encountered, obstetricians were seen as the most authoritative. The women also used professionals for advice before taking a course of action, for example, trying to become pregnant, exercising in pregnancy and stopping smoking. Professional advice was usually valued above that of family and friends, with the exception of Elise, whose sister was a health visitor. However Rosie saw value in the experiences other women had in childbearing. The greater knowledge of professionals was acknowledged by most and Tina voiced what was implied by others. 'You're coming to hospital because you feel they are the people that should know things that you, yourself, don't know.' Angela stated an unquestioning trust in her doctor, whereas Elise was prepared to use her own judgement: 'I have a good rapport with my GP, I would certainly take notice. I might well check it out somewhere else as well if it didn't sound right.'

Professionals may be rated according to perceived expertise or alternatively on closeness of personal relationship. Elise said 'The doctor's advice at clinic would carry more weight than that of the GP, because I see the GP as someone who deals with everything to a certain level and not particularly skilled in obstetrics. I would probably rate the midwife about similar to the GP or just below.' Jean said 'It really depends on the person giving the advice. If I was more familiar with the doctor, then I'd probably rather go with him, if I'd only just met the midwife.'

The style of advice-giving was likely to affect its acceptability. Respect for doctors' expertise did not necessarily mean slavish obedience. The women implied that they felt they had the right to make their own decisions about their lives. Angela, in spite of her trust in her doctor, clearly felt herself to be in charge of her life. She smoked and was aware of the dangers of smoking in pregnancy. She welcomed advice and appreciated respect from her doctor. 'He treated me as if I was sensible enough to be able to make that decision myself.' None of the women liked dictatorial advice-giving.

Health professionals have been encouraged to give health advice with regard to the cultural background of their clients. Here was an example of a client assuming that the advice she was being given to reduce her workload was affected by the doctor's cultural background. Sonia said 'The GP has kept on saying, you must give up work, but he is an Indian and I think he just doesn't believe you should try and juggle everything, so I take it more as a sort of culture thing, than a health thing'. Elise was confident in her own ability to use the system to her own advantage but recognized that others may be less well-equipped to do so. She implied, as did other women, that midwives were less intimidating than doctors. Feeling threatened or intimidated may prevent women from taking available opportunities to gain information and advice. Although most of the women attended antenatal classes, enjoyed them and gained from them, Rosie did not; 'I was asked to go, but I didn't, I was going to come for the "labour" antenatal class, but I'm so squeamish, so 'cos I couldn't find no one to come with me I wouldn't come, in case I passed out or got frightened.'

Although some personal advice was offered, it was more likely to be sought by the women. Much information was gleaned from written material, either given by professionals or found by the women themselves. Some professionals offered individual advice. Angela said 'It was my antenatal visit just before Christmas and the midwives were saying, have a great time, just be a bit sensible about alcohol'.

Written information was often given by professionals. *The Pregnancy Book* from the Health Education Authority was valued. A midwife may feel that when giving a standard bundle of information to a woman at the antenatal booking clinic she is giving information to a specific individual. However, the women in this study did not perceive this as personal advice. The women sought written information for themselves and seemed confident they were getting reliable information through commercial pregnancy literature, finding no conflicting advice. They implied they expected to take some of the initiative in information-gathering. They did not expect health professionals to probe to discover needs. Christine said 'I suppose these people just take it for granted that you should know'. There also seemed to be a feeling that constraints of money or time prevented professionals from offering a truly individual service. Only one woman felt that any attention had been paid to her mental well-being. Christine had left a violent partner, but did not seem to feel it was appropriate to discuss this. Rosie said she felt depressed and her response was similar.

Attitudes to media information

The general population is exposed to a great deal of health information through television, radio, newspapers and magazines. The attitudes of the women to this type of health advice varied. The women saw media advice as general and they exercised judgement as to whether it applied to them personally. They might also be prompted to enquire further about some media items. Media advice was more likely to be heeded if it was perceived to be authoritative, personally relevant and it reinforced personal experience or knowledge already held. However there was criticism of and scepticism about 'scares'. Some high-profile media coverage was remembered. Although it had been some 5 years since Edwina Currie, as Minister of Health, highlighted the problem of eggs as a source of *Salmonella* infection, she was remembered and quoted by three women.

Several women implied, and Tina stated, an increased interest in pregnancy-related health issues in the media. Angela implied and Elise made a direct statement about knowledge stored for future use: 'When the *Listeria* scare first came out, I wasn't planning a pregnancy but I thought that might affect me in the future and I read what I could about it'. If media advice relates to personal or family experience, the likelihood that it will be heeded is increased. Rosie said 'My brother's girlfriend, she drank all the way through her pregnancies and her little boys suffered from "fetal alcohol syndrome", that's what put me off'.

There was general criticism among the interviewees of the way health issues are presented in the media. Sensationalizing the information may cause women to ignore it and it was also criticized for possibly causing anxiety. Angela said 'Hearing it through the media, I think they always blow it out of proportion and so I tend not to bother.'

Two women made an interesting, but not very flattering analogy between health advice and media astrology. Diane commented 'I think just like your stars in the newspaper, it's so general as it's given out that you apply the bits you think you want to hear, don't you?' Angela said 'It's a bit like reading your horoscope, that's the way I tend to treat it, I always read it, but I don't take a lot of notice'.

Implications for health promotion

Opportunities for health promotion

The study demonstrated that opportunities for health education occurred but appeared not to have been exploited to the full. Interventions at any stage of a woman's life have the potential to influence the health of her future family. Pregnant women are presently asked about family health in order to assess pregnancy and fetal risks. It is suggested that the significance of lifestyle in relation to ill-health they have witnessed could be brought to the attention of pregnant women when discussing family health at the booking clinic. The workplace is one situation that could be exploited for health promotion to a greater extent. One might have expected the younger women in the study to have been exposed to health education in school. If they were, the lessons were certainly not remembered. More cooperation between health professionals and teachers could be of benefit. Participation in and enjoyment of a sport often begins at school and the health benefits of such activity could be reinforced by teachers. Eadie (1987) indicated that pleasure is a strong motivator for behaviour and the study confirmed this, especially where socially based exercise was concerned.

The general feeling from the study was of women who wished and expected to have control over the decisions which could influence health. The medical model of health was still fairly strongly in evidence in the women's stories and the medical profession was seen as the main arbiter of healthy pregnancy. There is scope for empowerment of women to enable them to place greater value on their own needs and wishes and have more involvement in decision-making.

Most of the women interviewed were happy to be pregnant and even those who had some ambivalent feelings about the pregnancy showed positive, protective and responsible feelings towards their babies. It would appear that it was the actual pregnancy rather than a desire to have a baby that caused them to become more health conscious and to make changes. This may explain some of the lack of enthusiasm for preconception care, and indeed only Elise sought such care. The concern for the baby and actual changes in health behaviour confirm pregnancy as a time when health education can be effective. Physical changes which lead to improvements, for example, when nausea reduces smoking in early pregnancy, could possibly be used to assist more long-term behaviour change. Pregnancy could be the trigger which activates previous health education for example, having learnt in the past that smoking was unhealthy, an attempt to give up or cut down may be made during pregnancy. Therefore information unheeded at the time it was received is not necessarily wasted. Many of the women in this sample felt a strong sense of responsibility for the baby as someone who was unable to protect himself or herself. This can be utilized in health education but should not be employed to the point of causing guilt or anxiety. Research by Condon and Hilton (1988) showed that where behaviour fell short of what their respondents desired, or what they perceived society expected of them, they tended to rationalize or justify their actions in order to lessen anxiety or possible criticism.

The women in this study did not appear to expect a detailed personal assessment of their needs but where they sought advice, that given by a trusted professional was likely to be given credence. The more highly educated and health-aware women made sure they received the information they felt they needed. A study by Rautava and Sillanpää (1991) highlighted the need for individual assessment for those women least aware of pregnancy health issues, who were also less likely to feel the need for information. Articulate women are most likely to get the best out of the system in which they find themselves. For women who experience difficulty in communicating because of language problems or disability, or whose youth or poor education puts them at a disadvantage, a number of measures can be taken to redress imbalances. Health promoters need to utilize all their skills in communication and may need specific training and up-dating on how to help disadvantaged women. They also need to be given time to do this job. Women themselves could be helped by specific measures, such as awareness or assertiveness programmes. Antenatal care can be carried out either in the women's homes, or in other venues where they could meet other women in a non-threatening atmosphere.

Two of the women in the study had needs which they did not see as falling within the remit of those who were caring for them. Both were feeling somewhat depressed and one saw the cause as her social problems. There was very little evidence in the study of professional interest in the mental well-being of any of these pregnant women. Those within the NHS having direct care of pregnant women have virtually no influence which could improve their social conditions. However there is scope for professionals to demonstrate more overt interest and support.

There was a hint in the study of the need for partners to be better informed. The women saw them in a protective, supporting role, but words like 'fear', 'anxiety' and 'worry' occurred frequently, and suggest that the partners could fulfil a supportive role more effectively and with more equanimity if they had better knowledge of childbearing and childrearing. In this study, where partners were not present, the mothers of the respondents fulfilled a similar supporting role. When a woman does not have a partner involved, it could be helpful to discover who is the most significant person in her life during the pregnancy and involve that individual as far as possible in her care. Support for the pregnant woman may then be enhanced. Aaronson (1989) highlights the importance of both perceived and received support in facilitating positive health behaviour in pregnancy and Haug *et al.* (1992) suggests partner support in stopping smoking is helpful.

The background to a woman's decision to breastfeed or not may stretch far back into her childhood. The accepted wisdom is that most women have made up their minds on their preferred method of feeding before pregnancy. This study showed that even those women apparently confirmed as 'anti-breastfeeding' may change. Comments from two women suggested they had retained some idea that breastfeeding was desirable but that only the reality of pregnancy allowed them to seriously contemplate it themselves. Most of the women displayed a need for education in breastfeeding, particularly those who were undecided. The one woman who had made a conscious, reasoned and apparently firm decision to bottle-feed admitted she had blocked out information about breastfeeding and it seems unlikely that she would be deflected from her resolve. However the midwife does have a responsibility to raise the issues with such women in a non-judgemental way, so choice is truly informed.

Health promotion is more likely to be effective if it starts from where the women are, rather than starting from where health promoters believe them to be. Professionals often complain of insufficient resources, including time, to do their job effectively. However, if time is not spent assessing needs, much well-meaning effort will be wasted. 'Lectures' are sometimes seen as a speedy way of imparting knowledge, but group work in parentcraft can be far more effective as the discussions can often show the group facilitator the particular needs of individuals and help the participants to discover hitherto unperceived needs.

Relationships with professionals

The valued features of professional support appeared to be correct advice perceived to be authoritative but non-dogmatic, given by people with whom the women had a good continuing personal relationship. It is difficult to form such a relationship if the pregnant woman attends an antenatal clinic and sees a different doctor or midwife at each visit. Power *et al.* (1989) highlighted the importance of reinforcement and personal interest when assisting pregnant women to stop smoking. It would seem good practice to ask those who said they were non-smokers, if they had recently stopped and offer support as appropriate. Where women in the sample rated the advice by different health professionals, obstetricians were the most highly rated, yet little positive health education was done by them. Two possible actions are suggested by this, either to attempt to increase the educator role of doctors or to increase the standing of others, particularly midwives. A third possibility having regard for the importance of individual assessment of needs is for greater liaison between members of any team of professionals caring for pregnant women.

Professionals would also do well to remember they can be intimidating to some clients. Midwives were seen by the women in the study as less intimidating but they were also seen as having a lower status than doctors. This suggests that midwives need to do more to raise their status in the eyes of pregnant women.

Several women had attended and enjoyed antenatal classes, the formal health education provision for pregnancy. Much work in recent years had led to improving the standards and accessibility of this provision. However, professionals must not consider health promotion is carried out only in such classes. Every contact with a pregnant woman should be seen as a potential health promotion opportunity.

It would appear that highly educated women are more likely to question the advice given by professionals, but this, of course, does not imply that the less well-educated accept and act on advice more readily. It does follow that professionals must be ready to explain and justify their advice.

Written information was seen as useful and important and reinforcement by professionals validates and emphasizes the health messages. This study supports the findings of Strychar *et al.* (1990) in which written material and doctors' advice dominated the resources used by the women.

The media, both newspapers and television, had some impact on the women in the study. Health 'scares' were, on the whole, treated sensibly, with neither panic reactions nor total disregard. However given the high value placed on professional personal advice and support, the study suggests that professionals should make themselves aware of what is in the media in order to have the full facts to hand.

Summary of key points

- In midwifery, health promotion and education should start from where the woman is. In order to find out this information the midwife should explore with each woman she cares for how health is defined, and to what degree she feels she has power over her health. This will help the midwife to discover how open or resistant each woman is to the various aspects of health promotion and to tailor her communication with the woman accordingly. If time is not spent assessing women's health needs, much well-meaning effort will be wasted.
- Lay definitions of health usually contain positive elements as well as negative ones in the form of absence of disease. People's definitions often reflect a medical model of disease causation and when medicine is seen as unable to explain and cure ill-health, for instance in some cases of cancer, fear is often demonstrated in the lack of medical control.

- Although health is sometimes seen by lay people as within individual control, for instance the effects of smoking, it does not necessarily follow that a smoker will stop smoking to improve their health chances. Such health behaviour has been attributed to socio-economic class differences by some researchers, the 'middle classes' being more likely to accept responsibility for ill-health caused by neglect, and the 'working classes' more likely to be fatalists who accept less self-responsibility for ill-health.
- Health may be regarded as desirable and an essential precondition for a full life, but health-enhancing behaviour will often be ignored if it conflicts with main life priorities such as pleasure and enjoyment.
- Semi-structured interviews with a small sample of women led to their comments being categorized as attitudes to health; attitudes to pregnancy and making changes; relationships with professionals; and attitudes to media information. Their comments, although not representative of the whole population, have many parallels with current literature about health beliefs, attitudes and behaviour.
- It would appear from this study and the literature that opportunities to promote health before and during pregnancy are not optimized. It is suggested that health education at school, the antenatal booking appointment and parent education sessions are good opportunities to explore health issues around childbearing and parenting.
- The women in this study appeared to be strongly influenced by the medical model of childbirth, seeing doctors as the main arbiters of a healthy pregnancy. There is continuing scope for empowerment of women to enable them to place greater value on their own needs and wishes, and have more involvement in decision-making.
- In this study it appeared that the actual pregnancy, rather than the desire to have a baby, caused the women to become more health conscious and to make changes. This has implications for preconception care and is one possible explanation of why, for instance, so few women take periconception folic acid supplements, despite its known advantages in the prevention of neural tube defects.
- Although health professionals have little if any influence over the social conditions of individual pregnant women there is scope for them to demonstrate more overt interest and support of women who live in trying circumstances.
- Health professionals must be ready to explain and justify their advice.

References

Aaronson, L.S. 1989: Perceived and received support: effects on health behaviour during pregnancy. *Nursing Research* 38(1), 4–9.

Allison, K.R. 1991: Theoretical issues concerning the relationship between perceived control and preventive health behaviour. *Health Education Research* 6(2), 141–51.

Blaxter, M. and Paterson, L. 1982: *Mothers and daughters: a three generation study of health attitudes and behaviour.* London: Heinemann Educational.

Calnan, M. 1987: *Health and illness, the lay perspective.* London: Tavistock.

Condon, J.T. and Hilton, C.A. 1988: A comparison of smoking and drinking behaviours in pregnant women: who abstains and why. *Medical Journal of Australia* 148, 381–5.

Eadie, D.R. 1987: Relationships between health and fitness and the implications for health education. *Health Education Research* 2(2), 81–91.

Haug, K., Aarø, L.E. and Fugelli, P. 1992: Smoking habits in early pregnancy and attitudes towards smoking among pregnant women and their partners. *Family Practice* 9(4), 494–9.

Herzlich, C. 1973: *Health and illness.* London: Academic Press.

Holt, J. 1984: *How children fail.* Harmondsworth: Penguin.

Pill, R. and Stott, N. 1982: Concepts of illness causation and responsibility; some preliminary data from a sample of working class mothers. *Social Science and Medicine* 16, 13–51.

Power, F.L., Gillies, P.A., Madeley, R.J. and Abbott, M. 1989: Research in an antenatal clinic – the experience of the Nottingham Mothers' Stop Smoking Project. *Midwifery* 5, 106–12.

Rautava, P. and Sillanpää, M. 1991: The effect of guidance on the knowledge level of expectant mothers seen at maternity health care clinics. *Hygie* 10(4), 12–17.

Strychar, I.M., Griffith, W.S. and Conry, R.F. 1990: The relationship among learning, health beliefs, alcohol consumption, and tobacco use of primigravidas. *Canadian Journal of Public Health* 81, 462–7.

Williams, R. 1983: Concepts of health: an analysis of lay logic. *Sociology* 17, 185–204.

12

Smoking and pregnancy: the role of midwives

Val Thomas

Promoting cessation for pregnant smokers is now seen as an integral part of the midwife's role as health promoter. The Health of the nation *in 1992 set a target for smoking reduction in the UK: 'In addition to the overall reduction in prevalence, at least 33% of women smokers to stop smoking at the start of their pregnancy by the year 2000' (Department of Health, 1992).*

Thirty-eight per cent of all mothers smoke before pregnancy. A quarter of those claim to quit during pregnancy, and of those who quit, half of them will start again within a month of the baby's birth. The Health Education Authority (HEA) has stated that one in three continue to smoke at some time during their pregnancy (Ford, 1994).

Midwives, smoking cessation and ethics

The first chapters of this book described various concepts of health and some philosophical difficulties that health education and health promotion pose for the midwife. Pregnant women who smoke raise many of these issues. As a medical fact, smoking is recognized as being unhealthy for mothers and their unborn children. However pregnant smokers may not share that perspective. They may not see quitting smoking as being one of their own felt 'health needs'. The felt health needs of an individual are a product of her own medical history and of her ethnic, cultural and social and family background.

Midwives are expected to give pregnant smokers information about the effects of smoking on pregnancy and help them make decisions about attempting to quit. The issue is a good example of how necessary it is for midwives to clarify their own beliefs and attitudes towards smoking. This applies equally to smokers and non-smokers. Many non-smokers believe smoking to be an evil, and take an evangelical approach to promoting the non-smoking message. On the other hand, midwives who smoke them-selves may feel hypocritical and uncomfortable when promoting the non-smoking message.

If midwives are aware of their own attitudes and beliefs and how they were formed, these can lead to greater understanding of the numerous influences on pregnant smokers. Midwives' acceptance that ultimately individual women must decide for themselves if they wish to quit smoking, will find self-exploration enables them to develop skills for helping women in this process. Any health promotion should be based on trying to understand the influences that shape beliefs and attitudes and providing the appropriate information and stimuli that lead to their reformulation.

With this understanding in their minds, midwives promoting smoking cessation should recognize that there are two distinct elements in any intervention process. It is the smoker herself who must take responsibility and control of her behaviour. This does not rest with midwives. The responsibility of health promoters is, by using their skills, to help individ-uals to change their behaviour.

Research and smoking cessation in pregnancy

The research into smoking and pregnancy and smoking cessation has concentrated on different aspects. These include the health risks, the demographics, the interventions and their outcomes and the cost benefits of promoting smoking cessation in pregnancy. This research has demon-strated that smoking and pregnancy is an issue that has a number of serious consequences and that midwives are in a position to address these problems.

The health risks of smoking and pregnancy

The health risks of smoking in pregnancy are well-researched and the ill-effects on the pregnancy and the unborn baby are well-documented. The HEA named the following conditions that the research associates with smoking in pregnancy (HEA, 1994):

- Smoking reduces fertility, and women who smoke may take longer to conceive than non-smokers.
- Smoking does affect male fertility.
- There is an increased risk of ectopic pregnancy among smokers.
- There is an increased risk of spontaneous abortion.
- Women who smoke during pregnancy are twice as likely to experience premature labour.
- Mean birthweight is decreased and the likelihood of low birthweight increased. Estimates vary amongst studies. Birthweight is reduced by an average of approximately 200 g and the proportion of low birthweight babies is approximately doubled by cigarette smoking.
- There is higher fetal, neonatal and perinatal mortality in children born to women who smoke. The higher risk to mortality is independent of various factors such as education and social class, which are also associated with mortality.

The effects of smoking after the birth continue:

- Sudden infant death syndrome (SIDS) has been associated with smoking antenatally or postnatally or both. Maternal smoking during pregnancy will usually be followed by postnatal smoking. There is also an independent increase in the risk of SIDS associated with partners who smoke.
- Passive smoking by infants and children also increases the risks of respiratory problems, asthma attacks and ear disease (glue ear).

Who smokes?

If midwives wish to help pregnant women to stop smoking it is important that they understand the influences that pregnant women are under. Although giving only a general picture, it is useful to look at the background of pregnant smokers. Again, midwives will recognize these pregnant smokers as they meet them frequently in their work. A review of the literature by Forrest *et al.* (1995) has found smoking in pregnancy to be associated with:

- lower social class,
- women of lower educational achievement,
- single, divorced or separated women,
- women under the age of 20,
- women who started to smoke when they were under 17 years of age,
- daily exposure to other people smoking at home,
- high parity,
- women who are white (other ethnic groups are less likely to smoke),
- the amount smoked at conception – heavier smokers are less likely to give up successfully.

The interventions

Studies of interventions designed to promote smoking cessation in pregnancy have taken place in a number of countries, including the UK. The interventions vary from briefly advising a pregnant smoker to stop smoking, to offering a planned programme of support. Overall advice about smoking cessation was found to be most effective when advice was given regularly in pregnancy and became integrated into routine antenatal care. O'Connor *et al.* in 1992 compared cessation rates between pregnant smokers receiving advice at their first antenatal visit with women who were merely referred to smoking cessation classes. The group receiving an intervention in the antenatal setting had two to three times higher rates of cessation at all follow-up periods. Another study by Sexton and Hebel in 1984 found that the impact on pregnant smokers of offering advice was greatest when it was repeated several times throughout pregnancy.

A number of studies indicate that the most effective interventions are those especially tailored to the pregnant woman. For example Hjalmarson *et al.* in 1991 found that 10.4 per cent of women stopped smoking when they received a specially designed self-help manual compared with a rate of 5.2 per cent for a group who were simply given an information sheet with the basic facts about pregnancy and smoking. A study by Ershoff *et al.* (1989) reported a cessation rate of 22 per cent when the information was in a series of booklets given throughout the pregnancy and the advice was especially tailored.

A study carried out in the UK at a Nottingham hospital focused upon interventions made by the midwifery staff. A pregnant smoker was given a 'designated midwife' to answer any questions and to provide friendly advice and encouragement at all antenatal visits, a carbon monoxide monitor was used by mothers to check their own progress and a specially written booklet was given along with the offer of self-help groups. Only 10 per cent of the women said that this programme had not had any effect. Among the effects described by the women were: made to think (42 per cent), 'Have a go' at cutting down (32 per cent) and helped to stop (10 per cent). The authors concluded that interventions that are simple, which show a personal interest in individual women and which encourage full women and partner participation are likely to gain the support and commitment of women and clinic staff. Midwives have a key role as the 'friendly encourager' (Power *et al.*, 1989).

The financial cost of smoking in pregnancy

Stopping smoking during pregnancy has a substantial impact on the health of the mother and the fetus. The most well-documented studies have been on smoking cessation and birthweight. For example Fox and colleagues in 1988 found that smoking cessation in pregnancy is associated with a 200–300 g increase in birthweight.

The financial costs of treating the consequences of smoking during pregnancy are high. Most studies have been made in the USA and indicate that the costs of treating interuterine growth retardation and prematurity in neonatal units are enormous. Immense savings can be made by smoking cessation interventions offered during pregnancy.

Marks *et al.* in 1990 made a cost benefit/cost effectiveness study of a smoking cessation intervention programme. They concluded, by making an analysis of the costs of caring for low birthweight babies in intensive care units, that for every $1 spent on intervention, $3.31 would be saved by decreasing the number of low birthweight babies requiring specialized long-term care. Windsor *et al.* (1993) found a cost-to-benefit ratio of $1 to $6.72 (low estimate) and $1 to $17.18 (high estimate). Studies are now being undertaken in the UK that are revealing a similar picture. Buck and Godfrey (1994) concluded that the cost of establishing a smoking cessation programme in pregnancy would be more than offset by the averted costs associated with the increased risks of low birthweight.

An economic analysis indicates that preventative interventions not only improve the health and well-being of mothers and their babies, but also are a means of preserving scarce funding resources.

Promoting smoking cessation

There are many different methods of promoting smoking cessation. There are the general control measures that provide information and affect sales and use of tobacco. These include regular increases in the real price of tobacco, a complete ban on all advertising, promotion and sponsorship, and the restriction of smoking in public places. Midwives and other health professionals are particularly well placed to promote the no-smoking message. This is because of pregnant women's opportunities. Individuals expect and respect the advice of health professionals, and those who use the health service are usually receptive to advice. The HEA (1993) has stated that users of the health service receive one-to-one advice which is considered to be effective in changing people's behaviour and this is reinforced by continuity of care and follow-up.

How can midwives effectively promote smoking cessation amongst pregnant smokers?

Research has shown that there are particular methods that midwives can use in their care of pregnant smokers. First, advice should be integrated into routine antenatal care. Secondly, pregnant women are more likely to give up smoking if they are advised to do so on several occasions, rather than just once. Thirdly West (1994) found the use of specially tailored written information for pregnancy was more effective than more generalized information.

Given the time constraints of the routine antenatal visit, how best may midwives make a short, sharp, effective intervention? There are a number of models that have been developed to help smokers quit. Models of behavioural change tend to be based on change in attitudes. Downie *et al.* (1996) for instance, describe attitudes as being central to health promotion as they tie together the individual's beliefs and feelings. Smoking behaviour depends on the smoker's attitudes to smoking. So these attitudes usually have to change before smoking behaviour changes.

Understanding why individuals hold beliefs and attitudes is extremely complicated. For example, various studies have shown that pregnant women who continue to smoke usually know of the dangers of smoking to themselves and their babies. A smoking and pregnancy tracking survey of 526 women carried out by the HEA in March 1993 (Ford, 1994) found that the majority (89 per cent) of pregnant women in the sample considered smoking to be harmful to their unborn child. Another study by Lucas (1994) of detailed analyses of women's beliefs about smoking in both early and late pregnancy also revealed that women generally accepted that smoking is detrimental to the unborn child. However, women who smoke during pregnancy believe that the complications of smoking are unlikely to happen to them.

Midwives will recognize these beliefs amongst pregnant smokers. Their formation is complex and reflects the individual background of each woman. By using a model of change (*see* Fig. 12.1) midwives can help themselves and pregnant smokers understand these processes. Pregnant smokers may then be helped to go on to reformulate their beliefs and attitudes about their own smoking behaviour.

The dynamics of the model are that behavioural change passes through a number of phases that usually represent attitudinal changes. These changes are usually gradual and may occur over months or years. In the model of smoking behaviour developed by the HEA (Fig. 12.1) these phases change from the person starting to think about change to the quitter and relapser (HEA, 1994).

Outside of the model is the 'contented smoker', the person who expresses no desire to quit. For example, a typical statement may be: 'I've smoked all my life and never had a day's illness, like my mother before me'. Pregnant smokers who hold this attitude have not yet started the process of change and may be quite resistant to even starting to think about quitting. Efforts are best concentrated upon women who have already entered the change process as these women are more likely to have future attitude and behavioural changes.

Thinking about change is seen as the first step towards quitting smoking. This is followed by making preparations to change, then by

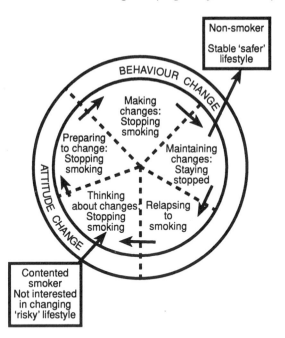

Figure 12.1 Model of attitude and behaviour change. Note: Professional help for pregnant women varies according to the smoker's position on the cycle of change. (Adapted from HEA, 1994. © Health Education Authority. Reproduced with kind permission)

making the changes, i.e. giving up. The non-smoking behaviour then has to be maintained, and there is always the possibility of relapse. Some people pass through this cycle many times, quitting and relapsing before staying as a non-smoker.

In using this type of model it is necessary to look at the woman holistically. What are the pressures that a woman experiences in her own existence that cause her to smoke? What are her own perceptions of the dangers of smoking and the benefits of giving up? Each woman will be different in terms of her dependence, and reasons for not quitting or in her determination to quit. For example some women live lives where their health is compromised by numerous factors. They might be unemployed, or living in poor social conditions. The dangers of smoking may not loom large against these pressures. More important to their health might be the perceived stress relief gained from smoking.

The skill of the health-promoting midwife is to understand these factors and to enable women to understand themselves. Through this process the midwife can help women identify why they smoke and why they would like to stop. However it is important that it is the pregnant smokers themselves who take responsibility for the process. The role of midwives is to facilitate and positively support women.

How to help pregnant smokers move through the cycle of change

A useful starting point for a midwife hoping to promote change in a pregnant smoker is to think of any personal behavioural changes. She may compare changes that she has made in response to a request or persuasion, with those that were a consequence of a conscious decision. She may then reflect on which types of changes have produced sustained behavioural changes.

Stimulating behavioural change is a skilful process. Communication skills are vitally important. Women who smoke are well aware that they will be 'advised' to quit smoking by their midwives. It is a sensitive issue and Lucas (1994) found in his study that guilt-producing advice is likely to increase some women's desire to continue smoking.

The model of attitude and behaviour change shown in Fig. 12.1 has been used as a basis for a training package devised by the HEA for health professionals helping pregnant women to quit. Health professionals who undertake this training will learn about the model and develop skills that will help them advise pregnant smokers in a way that will facilitate change. The approach is non-confrontational and exploratory. It is important that women do not feel that they are being subjected to an interrogation process. Open questions are used to raise issues such as 'What do you understand about the consequences of quitting?' The midwife should try to identify those women who are attempting to undergo behavioural change. The aim is to give information, advise and positively support women when they are making decisions about their smoking behaviour.

The following are the guidelines that the HEA training package gives for health professionals wishing to help pregnant smokers by using the model of change. They describe the approach for each stage of the model (HEA, 1994).

The contented smoker

- Decide to give second-order priority to smoking cessation work (but not other work) with this category of smoker.
- Correct any misinformation.
- Give information and advice if needed.
- Offer future support if wanted.
- Warn that the smoker will be asked again about quitting.

Thinking about change

- Exchange information. This should include:
  - (a) exploring the smoker's attitude to quitting, the pressures on her and her level of dependence;
  - (b) providing personally relevant information and correcting mis-information.
- Offer advice and guidance on stopping. Explore suitable possibilities of action that the woman might take, such as:
  - (a) taking regular breath tests to detect carbon monoxide;
  - (b) keeping a smoker's diary to record her smoking habits and to detect crucial smokes (i.e. when she is most likely to smoke), whether it was really needed and how much it was really enjoyed;
  - (c) identifying and jotting down all the benefits of stopping and pinning them up in a prominent place in the home;
  - (d) describing to herself the positive life she would like to have as a non-smoker;
  - (e) designating part of her home as a no-smoking area;
  - (f) finding out where the nearest smokers' clinic is.
- Provide encouragement.
- Offer follow-up support.
- Tell the smoker that she will be asked again about quitting.
- Ensure postnatal contact about smoking.

Preparing to change/Making changes

- Repeat or develop an exchange of personally relevant information.
- Advise and guide. Explore possible actions the woman could take (concentrating on 'dos', not 'don'ts'), such as:
  - (a) declaring a date a 'quit smoking' day to give up and telling family and friends;
  - (b) ditching the apparatus, getting rid of cigarettes, ashtrays, lighters;
  - (c) aiming to quit completely, not just reduce (reducers inhale more; quitters are likely to relapse at first but eventually do give up);
  - (d) getting support from family and friends, ex-smokers or Quit-line;
  - (e) distracting herself (especially on her personal 'quit smoking' day) and doing something different from when she used to smoke most;
  - (f) avoiding other smokers.
- Offer practical help where appropriate.
- Encourage.
- Offer follow-up support with yourself (ensure you can be contacted) or suggest other professional support.

Maintaining changes

- Ensure postnatal contact with women who have quit smoking in pregnancy.
- Repeat postnatal contact with women who have quit smoking in pregnancy (70 per cent restart smoking).
- Advise and guide. Explore possibilities of action that the woman could take, such as:
  - (a) dealing with today, concentrating on one day at a time;
  - (b) developing real alternatives and new activities;
  - (c) rewarding herself with the money that she saves;
  - (d) eating sensibly and taking appropriate physical exercise;
  - (e) detecting her withdrawal symptoms and being aware that the feelings are temporary. Severe symptoms occur in a minority only.
- Offer practical help where appropriate.
- Provide encouragement.
- Offer follow-up support with yourself or suggest other professional support.

Relapsing into smoking

- Exchange personally relevant information.
  - (a) Ensure that the smoker understands that relapsing is normal and provides useful learning.
  - (b) Help the smoker to explore the reasons why she relapsed.
  - (c) Identify the smoker's current position on the cycle of stopping (she may be resting; not 'thinking' about stopping).
  - (d) Advise and guide according to the smoker's current position on the cycle.
- Offer practical help.
- Provide encouragement.
- Offer future support or suggest alternative professional support.
- Warn that she will be asked again about quitting.

Summary of key points

- This chapter illustrates some of the basic principles of health promotion and how they may be employed to address some of the serious dangers to the health of pregnant women and their children. It is based on the premise that health promotion is about accepting that individuals make their own health choices based on their own personal experience of the world. Midwives may help pregnant women clarify their choices and decide how best they might adopt healthier behaviour within the constraints of their own environment.

- It presents the research that supports interventions designed to promote smoking cessation among pregnant women. This research demonstrates the health and cost benefits of smoking cessation during pregnancy. It also identifies interventions that have been found to be among the most effective in helping women to stop smoking. These should be started at antenatal booking and sustained throughout pregnancy. They should be specially tailored to individual women and be offered in the form of friendly, sympathetic advice.
- A model developed by the Health Education Authority from the work of researchers that helps midwives effectively work with pregnant smokers is described. It is designed to help midwives encourage and support pregnant smokers to stop smoking.
- Case histories are included to provide examples for midwives wanting to develop appropriate intervention techniques for helping pregnant smokers stop smoking (*see* Exercise 12.1).
- Midwives are particularly well-placed to help pregnant smokers improve and maintain the health of themselves and their babies. The statement that each pregnancy has its individual characteristics that the midwife must address, may also be applied to the pregnant smoker. The HEA model provides a tool for midwives to interpret the individual's characteristics of pregnant smokers, to encourage, support and help them to stop smoking.
- More information about smoking cessation may be obtained from the HEA, local health promotion departments or Quitline (London), tel. 0800 002200.

EXERCISE 12.1   Helping pregnant smokers

Below are three profiles of pregnant smokers. Imagine that you are in an antenatal consultation and wish to give some advice on smoking. How would you approach and raise the issue of smoking to identify the position of each woman on the cycle of change, and her beliefs about smoking? How would you help each woman and her midwife understand her beliefs and attitudes? What support and advice would you give the woman?

Case A
Josie is a 31-year-old mother of three children between the ages of 9 and 4. She is accidentally pregnant with her fourth child. She is university educated, but married on graduating and became pregnant shortly after starting her career. She worked after the birth of her first child but stopped after the second. She has a supportive partner, who does not smoke and few financial worries. She smokes 10–15 cigarettes a day, has given up twice before during her first two pregnancies, but relapsed shortly after the births.

Case B

Angela is 17 years old, and pregnant for the first time. She is unemployed and lives with her mother. The father of the child is her boyfriend Rick, also aged 17, who works in a supermarket. He is supportive but unable to contribute much financially. Angela's mother says she can only give her limited support as she has three other children and is a widow. Angela and her mother smoke but Rick does not.

Case C

Frances is 23 years old and works as a sales assistant in a fashion store. She also works as a part-time model. She married when she was 21 years old and this is her first pregnancy. Although it is a planned pregnancy, Frances intends to return to work after the birth. Her husband John is a salesman and they do not have any financial worries. Both Frances and John smoke approximately 10 cigarettes per day. Frances has never tried to quit, but John is a relapsed smoker.

References

Buck, D. and Godfrey, C. 1994: Helping smokers give up. Guidance for purchasers on cost effectiveness. London: HEA.

Department of Health 1992: *The health of the nation*. London: HMSO.

Downie, R.S., Tannahill, C. and Tannahill, A. 1996: *Health promotion: models and values*. Oxford: Oxford University Press.

Ershoff, D.H., Mullen, P.D. and Quinn, V.P. 1989: A randomized trial of a serialized self-help smoking cessation program for pregnant women in an HMO. *American Journal of Public Health* 79(2), 182–7.

Ford, K. 1994: Campaign overview. In *Health Education Authority (HEA) Smoking and Pregnancy Conference*. London: HEA, 8–9.

Forrest, D., Horsley, S., Roberts, E. and Barrow, S. 1995: Factors relating to smoking in pregnancy in the North Western Region. *Journal of Public Health Medicine* 17(2), 205–10.

Fox, N.L., Sexton, M.J. and Hebel, J.R. 1988: Smoking cessation and weight gain during pregnancy: effects on birth weight. *Teratology* 37(5), 457.

HEA (Health Education Authority) 1993: *Giving up smoking: does the patient education work?* London: HEA.

HEA 1994: *Helping pregnant smokers quit, training for health professionals*. London: HEA.

Hjalmarson, A.I.M., Hahn, L. and Svanberg, B. 1991: Stopping smoking in pregnancy: effect of a self-help manual in controlled trial. *British Journal of Obstetrics and Gynaecology* 98, 260–4.

Lucas, K. 1994: Attitudes and beliefs: the mothers' point of view. In *HEA Smoking and Pregnancy Conference*. London: HEA, 44–50.

Marks, J.S., Koplan, J.P., Hogue, C.J. and Dalmat, M.E. 1990: A cost benefit cost-effectiveness analysis of smoking cessation for pregnant women. *American Journal of Preventative Medicine* 6(5), 282–9.

O'Connor, A.M., Davies, B.L., Dulberg, C.S. *et al.* 1992: Effectiveness of a Pregnancy Smoking Cessation Program. *Journal of Obstetric, Gynaecological and Neonatal Nursing* 21(5), 385–92.

Power, F.L., Gillies, P.A., Madeley, R.J. and Abbott, M. 1989: Research in an antenatal clinic – the experience of the Nottingham Mothers' Stop Smoking Project. *Midwifery* 5(3), 106–12.

Sexton, M. and Hebel, J. 1984: A clinical trial of change in maternal smoking and its effect on birth weight. *Journal of the American Medical Association* 251(7), 911–15.

West, R. 1994: Interventions to reduce smoking among pregnant women. In *HEA smoking and pregnancy, guidance for purchasers and providers.* London: HEA, 9–29.

Windsor, R.A., Lowe, J.B., Perkins, L.L. *et al.* 1993: Health education for pregnant smokers: its behavioural impact and cost benefit. *American Journal of Public Health* 83(2), 201–6.

Further reading

HEA 1997: *Action on smoking and pregnancy: an information pack to help midwives, health visitors and practice nurses deal with smoking and pregnancy issues.* London: HEA.

13

Sexual health promotion

Maggie McNab

This chapter concentrates on various aspects of sexual health, how it relates to midwifery practice and the important contribution midwives can make in promoting sexual health. Sexual health promotion can be an exciting and challenging area of work. In common with health promotion in general, it involves taking account of various dimensions and concepts. It may be described as having physical, mental, emotional, social, spiritual and societal components (Ewles and Simnett, 1995). Sexual health crosses into all these areas which are interrelated and interdependent. It is not restricted to control of infections and it plays an important part in the health of individuals and communities.

Midwifery is tied closely to sexual activity, sexuality and sexual health. Conception is achieved by sexual intercourse and/or contact with, or exchange of, sexual body fluids and thenceforward the call for midwifery and obstetric services. Midwives, nurses and doctors meet a huge diversity of women with a multitude of needs and experiences: women in single-sex relationships who may choose to conceive by donor insemination, women who have vastly differing cultural and religious beliefs, younger women, older women, women with disabilities, well women and those who live with chronic ill-health. Sensitivity and awareness in a wide variety of situations is expected, both by the profession and by the public being cared for. Integrating sexual health promotion into midwifery practice can enhance and enrich the quality of care given.

Health promotion and sexual health promotion

Strategies for promoting health vary and it is noted in Chapter 5 of this book that there are probably over a hundred different approaches to health education and health promotion to choose from (Rawson, 1992). Some methods focus on information-giving, some rely on screening mechanisms, some stress individual behaviour modification and some of the broader approaches incorporate social, economic and fiscal policy and social and environmental changes. Defining, planning and employing different strategies have different effects on the outcomes, so it helps if there is some clarity about the aim of any health promotion exercise (Aggleton, 1992; Downie *et al.*, 1996).

Midwives may have access to abundant information about HIV and sexual health but such information is not very helpful or useful by itself. Many health professionals and others assume that people will change behaviour if they are aware of factors which contribute to ill-health. However, it is now widely accepted that although raising levels of information may increase knowledge and understanding, it is not suffi-cient to alter or make changes to health-related behaviour. Those who seek to promote sexual health within their practice need opportunities to explore some of their own professional attitudes, cultural influences or personal prejudices and time to reflect on how any knowledge might be used to enhance behaviour change by themselves or their clients. They also need to be given opportunities to consider the impact of other external influences, such as social isolation, unemployment, lack of trans-port, poor access to health and welfare services, cultural norms and family pressures, which may have strong, influential forces. Tones *et al.* (1990) argue that the issue of empowerment is a strong influencing factor for health promotion and that it enhances individuals, groups and communities to have control over different aspects of their lives. When involved in sexual health promotion it may be useful for midwives to consider different power relationships and, in particular, women's ability to be assertive. Men are often seen to have power over women (Richard-son, 1987; Doyal *et al.*, 1994) and how this affects women's ability to be assertive when trying to achieve safer sex may be an important factor.

Health promotion strategies based on individual responsibility are limited and need to be employed with broader based community initia-tives and political action. Broader approaches in midwifery may include establishing policies and strategies within the workplace which raise the level of support for sexual health promotion. These could include some creative action by midwives to establish truly health promoting services with and for the local communities, which are sensitive and responsive to the people midwives work with. Many of the approaches adopted by health promoters will be dictated by their role and function (Naidoo and

Wills, 1994). However, a knowledge of different approaches to health education and the wider concept of health promotion may be valuable when midwives and any others working in the broader field of health are considering how to make a positive contribution to sexual health promotion.

Sexual health promotion and HIV prevention work by Aggleton and Homans (1988) outline four main models incorporating different approaches. These are reported as being concerned primarily with information-giving, self-empowerment, community orientation and social change. This is a broad framework which encompasses various strategies and bears some similarity to the Ottawa Charter for Health Promotion (WHO, 1986b) which outlined the need to develop personal skills; enable, mediate and advocate; create supportive environments; strengthen community action and reorient health services.

Sexual health promotion impacts on both professional and personal lives. It is often regarded as a sensitive and personal issue which some find difficult to discuss overtly within the context of their work. The English National Board for Nursing, Midwifery and Health Visiting have issued guidelines (ENB, 1994) to encourage good practice in the teaching of sexual health education and training. The contributors acknowledge that sexual health and sexuality are important issues and that

> there is a delicate interface between the 'professional' and the 'personal'. Practitioners, managers, students and educationalists are also husbands, wives, lovers, partners, heterosexual, homosexual, lesbian, bisexual, in love, out of love, celibate, sexually active, sexually inactive – and have a whole range of sexual desires, beliefs, difficulties and fulfilments.

Sexual health and sexuality

Sexual health has been defined variously by different agencies and individuals. Positive definitions focus on being at ease with sexuality, enjoyment of sexual activity, making informed choices, personal and community empowerment, fulfilling relationships, planning of fertility and freedom from disease and abuse. Other definitions concentrate more on disease prevention and the avoidance of problems. Two of the better known definitions are summarized below. They outline many aspects of sexual health where midwives could and do contribute positively with individuals and communities.

The World Health Organization statement (WHO, 1986a) outlined three key elements of sexual health as:

- a capacity to enjoy and control sexual and reproductive behaviour in accordance with a social and personal ethic;
- freedom from fear, shame, guilt, false beliefs and other psychological factors inhibiting sexual response and impairing relationships;

- freedom from organic disorders, diseases and deficiencies that interfere with sexual and reproductive functions.

The International Programme Advisory Panel of the International Planned Parenthood Federation (IPPF, 1994) reviewed policy documents and discussion papers and issued statements endorsing their belief that:

1. Sexual health refers to somatic, as well as to emotional, intellectual and social aspects of sexuality.
2. People should have full knowledge of sexuality, its potentials and risks.
3. Sexuality is a positive force in human beings; the prevention of risks involved is not an end in itself, but together with freedom from psychological and physical problems is a requirement to take full advantage of its positive potential.
4. The concept of sexual health should not be rigidly applied; its meaning and scope depend on individual, social and cultural conditions.

In 1992 the British government published *The health of the nation* white paper which is a strategy document for health in England (Department of Health, 1992). Equivalent white papers were published for Scotland, Northern Ireland and Wales. These documents acknowledged that 'good personal and sexual relationships can actively promote health and well-being' (p. 92). Emphasis was placed on the importance of prevention of illness and the need to improve and maintain health, thereby not to lay focus on health care and the treatment of illness. Midwifery already has a firm footing within the health arena as most of the work has a focus on well-being and maintaining health, so it can and should provide a lead in promoting the public health.

HIV/AIDS (human immunodeficiency virus/acquired immune deficiency syndrome) and sexual health were selected as one of five key priority areas. Objectives and main targets for action were set. The objectives included:

- to reduce the incidence of HIV infection;
- to reduce the incidence of other sexually transmitted diseases;
- to reduce the number of unwanted pregnancies; and
- to ensure the provision of effective family planning services for those people who want them.

The main targets included detail about the desire to reduce:

- the incidence of gonorrhoea among men and women aged 15–64,
- the rate of conception amongst the under-16s,
- the percentage of injecting drug misusers who report sharing injecting equipment.

It is of interest to note that infection by gonorrhoea is used as one of the markers of unsafer sexual practices because symptoms of gonococcal infection are rapid whereas the time interval between infection with HIV and any symptoms is longer, often months and years rather than days or weeks. Likewise, the rate of pregnancy can be used as an indicator of unprotected sexual intercourse.

Since the advent of HIV infection and AIDS the importance of sexual health has become more pronounced and evident. Health services, local authorities, the voluntary sector, the education sector and the users of services are charged to work together with the government to meet the targets (Department of Health, 1992). However, those who work directly within the field of health are often seen to be most likely, and are considered to be better able, to take a lead in HIV prevention and sexual health promotion. This was supported in a study of women working in various agencies representing the statutory health services, local authorities and the voluntary sectors, in the field of sexual health and HIV prevention (McNab, 1993).

Midwives are well placed to make positive impacts on sexual health promotion and HIV prevention as their unique work provides the scope to build close personal relationships with women and their families. Opportunities for sexual health promotion are available pre-pregnancy, antenatally, during delivery and postpartum, in hospital and when visiting homes. The contacts may vary from one-to-one consultations in private to shared discussion with groups in parentcraft classes. Some opportunities will be presented by the midwife and some by those in her care. Midwifery services keep a close involvement throughout the pregnancy and postnatally and sometimes by working in the same geographical area midwives may develop a supportive rapport with the extended family. Midwives, nurses and health visitors are now expected to contribute to a broad range of initiatives within the arena of public health (Department of Health, 1993a, 1995a) and opportunities to develop services to meet the needs of women and their families are encouraged (Department of Health, 1993b; RCN, 1995). Any such political action or reorientation of services will demand professional support and integration into the service contracts for adequate support and funding.

Sexuality is concerned with the state and quality of being sexual (Collins, 1992) and it relates to 'complex and dynamic interactions between the capacity for desire, pleasure, imagination and communication and the mores of the societies in which we live' (Armstrong and Gordon, 1992). Personal attitudes about sexuality vary enormously and there is no standard guideline for health professionals or others. Rather it is for the individual to explore her own beliefs and to consider how they impact on both personal and professional responses. What is the range of accepted and non-accepted forms of behaviour, how do they affect attitudes to clients and how do these inform responses and affect subsequent communication? Such an exploration may include considering a number of different activities and identifying whether or not an activity or behaviour has any value, either personally or for others. For example, an individual midwife may prefer to be in a monogamous relationship but may think that having multiple partners is all right for others. Other examples of diversity in behaviour might include: having sex within or outside of marriage, being heterosexual or homosexual, having sex with another person or using sex toys, having sex in public places or only at home, having oral, anal or vaginal sex, having sex in order to have children or with no intention of getting pregnant (Armstrong and Gordon, 1992).

Formal sexual health training courses for health workers usually include comprehensive discussion on activities and language, where the participants are encouraged to become familiar and conversant with a broad range of practices and terminology. Such training may provide opportunities for reflection about personal attitudes and feelings and the impact of varying cultural and religious influences and should be recommended for all staff in order to influence and contribute towards good-quality service delivery. Time spent considering broad sexual issues may prepare an individual practitioner for better contact with the wider society and diverse community when working. It may also encourage ideas for implementing personal action plans and for individuals to exert pressure on services to address sexual health constructively within the workplace through practice and policy.

The use and meaning of the language and jargon readily employed in day-to-day conversation is an important consideration for sexual health promotion. For example, what do we mean by 'sex' or 'having sex'? How this may be interpreted relies on the understanding of the individual. This was illustrated to the author recently during history-taking in the setting of a family planning clinic when a young woman denied that she could have a positive pregnancy test because she had not had 'sex'. She divulged that she had been practising oral sex, anal intercourse and body rubbing in the genital area but had not had penetrative vaginal sex. In this instance it is significant that she believed that she had not 'had sex'. For most women 'having sex' will mean penetrative vaginal intercourse but for many it will involve a variety of different activities and some clarity is useful when 'safer sex' is on the agenda.

So, what do we mean by 'safer sex'? Is it merely linked to the use of condoms? If so, how knowledgeable are practitioners about their availability and the correct use of condoms and how well is this information shared? Is time taken to discuss the fact that the efficacy of the rubber is rapidly eroded when placed in contact with any oils and fat-based products? This is an important factor with the increasing popularity in the use of body massage oils and also when considering vaginal and anal lubricants. It may be especially important after delivery when resuming sexual intercourse may be assisted by some form of lubrication after episiotomy or when experiencing vaginal dryness. It is worth checking with the manufacturer before use, if there is any doubt about whether any preparations are water or oil-based. For instance, some pessaries for use in the treatment of vaginal thrush or candidiasis are not suitable for use with condoms but there are other preparations which are thought to be safe (Szarewski and Guillebaud, 1994). Safer sex may be better defined as any sexual activity which avoids an exchange of body fluids. If safer sex is to be broader than the use of condoms how can we develop conversations about safer sex, about sexual intercourse and sexuality? Training is an essential requirement in order to enhance development with work of this nature.

Empathizing with clients is important in midwifery and in other health care services and it is essential for good communication within the field of sexuality. Clients or service users will come from widely ranging experiences and expectations which will make certain demands on midwifery services. For instance, if a woman in a single-sex relationship is expecting her partner to accompany her in labour the midwife can make a positive contribution at this time if she is empathetic and supportive. She could also play an important part with all parents in broadening public perspectives about sexual stereotyping which often starts immediately after the birth, or before the birth, when the sex of the baby is determined.

HIV and AIDS

AIDS was first reported in the USA in 1981 and the virus, now known as HIV, was first identified as the causative agent in 1983. Initially it was thought to be a disease which only affected gay men but the realization that it could be transmitted through blood transfusion drew widespread attention from the media and brought about education and services for the wider public.

Transmission of the virus is by three main routes: through unprotected sexual intercourse, from an infected mother to her baby during pregnancy, birth and breastfeeding, and through infected blood or tissue transfer, including the sharing of needles and other injecting equipment by those using intravenous drugs. Infection attributed to HIV is steadily increasing and is thought to be the leading cause of death for women and men between 20–40 years of age in many cities in America, sub-Saharan Africa and Western Europe, including Britain (Panos, 1990). World wide the primary route of infection is by heterosexual intercourse. Despite advances in treatments there is slim likelihood of a cure at the moment, so it is imperative that prevention has a high priority.

In Britain, the proportion of newly diagnosed cases of HIV through sexual intercourse between men and women is steadily rising; from 8 per cent in 1989 to 19 per cent in 1996 (Public Health Laboratory Service, Communicable Disease Surveillance Centre, 1996). The Department of

Health (1995) issued a review of the government's HIV health promotion strategy, which states a commitment to continued maintenance of awareness in HIV in the general population. It also places emphasis on developing national and local health promotion directed towards targeted areas. Included in the list of identified groups are 'men and women who travel to, or have family links with, high prevalence countries where the predominant mode of transmission is sex between men and women, for example in sub-Saharan Africa'. It notes that there may be particular issues for women who may have male sexual partners in other groups chosen to be targeted like bisexual men and injecting drug users. This maintains emphasis and opportunities for midwives to take a pro-active role in HIV prevention and sexual health promotion and not just address the other important areas of care and treatment of those women known to be infected by HIV. This can be done by integrating health promotion into everyday discussions, practices and policies. Often staff are unaware of women who are HIV positive. A British study of pregnant women established that only 17 per cent of women from south-east England who tested HIV positive were identified before delivery, compared with 68 per cent in Scotland (Ades *et al.*, 1993).

Midwifery staff are well placed individually and professionally to become involved in sexual health promotion and also HIV prevention. This facet of the work and service delivery may be approached variously, at best in ways which are comfortable for the practitioners and the client. The evolving strategy (Department of Health, 1995b) will demand careful handling to avoid discriminatory practices if future action plans intend to stress activity with particular groups of the population. Discrimination will be avoided in those midwifery centres which have policies of offering everyone antenatal HIV testing which provides an opportunity to discuss transmission, and prevention, of infections.

Other sexually transmitted infections (STIs)

There are a large number of STIs which affect about a million men and women in Britain every year. Those affected come from all cultures, beliefs and economic levels. There is a large prevalence amongst teenagers and young adults. The situation is not helped by society's attitudes to sexuality and sexual behaviours. There is still great shame and fear of rejection about sexually transmitted infections, conversation remains restricted and some sexual activities are condemned so such infections are difficult to treat and control.

The list of STIs includes gonorrhoea and non-gonococcal genital infections (NGGI), such as chlamydia, trichomoniasis, genital warts or papillomavirus, genital herpes, syphilis, viral hepatitis, candidiasis, otherwise known as monilia or thrush, molluscum contagiosum, pubic lice and other infections which are rarely seen in Britain (Llewellyn-Jones, 1990). Further detail and statistical data are available from medical publications like the *British Medical Journal* and the *British Journal of Venereal Diseases*. Information may also be obtained from the Public Health Laboratory Service and a local profile can be obtained from genito-urinary medicine (GUM) services and other local public health services. Most infections can be treated and cured but some can have long-term effects and some can have a harmful effect on an unborn baby if treatment is not sought and made available. In the short term, many infections may affect the pleasure of any sexual contact and in the long term some may affect the fertility of both men and women.

Midwifery and other health services are familiar with the importance of the treatment and are conversant with the medical aspects of sexually transmitted infection. Pregnancy is largely regarded as a happy event and it may not be easy for us to discuss or disclose information about sexually transmitted infections. Many midwives are familiar with the shocked realization felt by a partner when told of a previously undiagnosed infection, 'How could I be infected? I've only had one partner for five years ...! Oh, not my partner ...?' Public understanding of STIs is generally thought to be poor (Health Education Authority, 1994) so it is essential to highlight primary prevention messages and to collaborate well with local services and referral agencies. *The health of the nation* (Department of Health, 1992) includes emphasis on the need to reduce the incidence of sexually transmitted infections. If individual practitioners are knowledgeable about the local services, and better still have visited personally in order to familiarize themselves with local services, such as the local GUM clinics, they will be better acquainted with the personnel, the local services and the locations and thus be better placed actively to encourage colleagues and clients to visit when in need of advice or treatment. A woman diagnosed as having gonorrhoea may experience a vast range of emotions and need a lot of support to cope with the information and the necessary treatment. She will be better able to do this if the midwife is well prepared to help her.

Family planning

Family planning issues, including fertility awareness, preconception care, psychosexual counselling, termination of pregnancy and contraception are important for the midwife and those in her care. Discussion on these topics can often be developed to foster broader debate about sexual health and to encourage referral to specialist counselling and treatment agencies when required.

Contraceptive consultation is commonly undertaken after childbirth and has become integrated into the holistic care of the mother. Other opportunities for discussion about contraception choices and sexual health may arise during booking and care when conversations are expanded. Topics may include detail about feelings towards the pregnancy, whether or not the pregnancy was planned, the relationship of the woman with her partner, if she has one, sexual enjoyment or difficulty and the intended family size. There are numerous methods available which prevent pregnancy and some, like the male and female condom, also protect against HIV infection and other STIs. Some of the more progressive midwifery services are now funded to supply free condoms to all women. Some contraceptive methods, such as the combined pill or the emergency postcoital pill which contain oestrogen, are not recommended for women who are breastfeeding. The choice of method is highly personal and the midwife may be asked to help women to decide. She will do this well if she is informed and has explored her own personal and professional attitudes and beliefs. A sound knowledge of some of these factors will enable her to provide guidance and advice which is sensitive to the needs of the individual and not biased by personal feelings.

Family planning choices are wide and various. Not all methods will suit all people and a method thought to be satisfactory for a period of time may need to be changed because of side-effects or change of circumstances. Great sensitivity and flexibility is needed on the part of the practitioner when guiding the woman or couple towards an acceptable and reliable method of choice. Detail can be sought from family planning practitioners and specialist services as well as in various dedicated texts on contraception and family planning which are readily available from local Health Authorities, Health Education or Health Promotion Services, the Family Planning Association, Brook Advisory Centres, the Catholic Marriage Advisory Council and from many good libraries and bookshops. Comprehensive training courses, like the ENB 901 – Family Planning, are available for health professionals, and regular updating days are held to maintain a current awareness for a range of practitioners, including midwives.

The health of the nation (Department of Health, 1992) highlighted the importance of reducing the number of unwanted pregnancies. As previously noted, the need to target effort at reducing the rate of conceptions amongst adolescents, particularly the under-16s, was highlighted. Studies of young people reveal that the age of first sexual intercourse is declining (Wellings *et al.*, 1994) and there is often poor understanding about contraception and reluctance to seek contraceptive advice (Thomas, 1996). Midwives may be able to create opportunities to encourage uptake of services by working with community organizations, families and young people to ensure that there is an increased awareness, that consultation confidentiality is assured and that condoms, pills and other methods are readily available and free of charge. There may also be opportunities to work as advocates for young people and to exert pressure, particularly at a local level, to ensure that such services are supportive and sensitive.

Evaluation of practice area

During recent specialist training in HIV awareness and sexual health promotion the author found very differing standards of midwifery practices, beliefs and policies. Some individual midwives and support staff are well-acquainted with the facts, have explored their personal and professional influence and impact and have involved themselves with interagency work, referrals to specialist agencies and creative broad-based sexual health promotion. Others are denying any role or active involvement with sexual health promotion outside those direct tasks of midwifery concerned with antenatal care of the mother, safe delivery of the baby and immediate care prior to discharge into the community.

Likewise, some midwifery services are showing exemplary practice in advertising an interest in sexual health to their clientele, by including information leaflets with the first contact letter and ensuring that the first consultation includes various aspects of sexual health promotion. Discussion about the local and national services available is encouraged to enhance care and education and challenge prejudicial practices. Some are employing specialist staff to assist the process of HIV prevention and sexual health promotion to achieve a high profile so that good standards and quality are considered. Others are maintaining a low profile in sexual health promotion, are slow to encourage the involvement and assistance of outside agencies and continue to employ discriminatory practices. Encouragement by management, financial support and further training needs to be prioritized and established in such areas.

The United Kingdom Central Council for Nursing, Midwifery and Health Visiting (UKCC, 1994) issues regular, updated guidelines for good practice which remind nurses, midwives and health visitors about their Code of Professional Conduct. These stress that practitioners should act 'always in such a manner as to promote and safeguard the interests and well-being of patients and clients'. Support needs to be provided where any practices seem to be at odds with this and subsequently fail to provide good standards of equality within service provision.

Within the area of infection control there is a particular challenge because discrepancy can arise between the requirements recommended from different departments and services. An example of this is provided by the guidelines written for midwives (UKCC, 1994) which cite that 'all blood and body fluids pose a potential infection risk and appropriate precautions must be taken'. The guidelines reinforce the responsibility to maintain good clinical practice in all situations 'irrespective of their serological status and any knowledge they may have of the serological status of their patients'. In order to provide a service which is non-discriminating this may be interpreted as assuming that everyone poses a potential risk and therefore should be treated the same. This immediately presents a problem in some service areas where different guidelines require that known infectious waste, for instance where someone has tested positive to HIV, is labelled differently from other waste materials. Creative service policies and procedures can be locally installed and put into practice to assist in redressing such obvious imbalances.

The author's recent discussions with midwives revealed that some are still not convinced of the need to employ recommended universal precautions and do not see the need to wear protective eye covering when delivering a woman regarded unlikely to pose any risk of infection. The same midwives were not opposed to following the recommended guidelines when caring for someone known to be infectious, thus establishing open discriminatory and potentially unsafe practice. Similar practice was also found in several studies reported in the midwifery and medical press (Willy *et al.*, 1990; Kabukaba and Young, 1992; Sharp *et al.*, 1993). HIV (and many other infections) does not discriminate and many women will be unknowingly infected (Ades *et al.*, 1993).

There is much that can be gained by greater involvement in sexual health promotion by midwifery and allied services which are well placed to make a positive impact. However, good support and adequate preparation for extending roles in this area will be needed. It is recognized that sexual health is an important component of the general health and well-being of individuals and societies (Department of Health, 1992). It is also acknowledged that there is some sensitivity between personal issues and professional areas of responsibility within sexual health.

With regard to HIV and AIDS there seem to be two distinct issues for midwifery and those services allied to midwifery. One addresses the infection itself and how it may affect the woman and her baby, their treatment and care; the other is how to develop the role of the midwife towards greater impact on prevention of infection and the broader aspects of sexual health promotion. There is inevitably some overlap and where service providers meet women affected directly by the virus an awareness of the many considerations and difficulties that HIV poses will be essential. It is important to secure opportunities for primary prevention throughout every service area.

In order to fully utilize the opportunities presented towards improving sexual health in the community, midwifery services need to ensure that access to current information is available. This includes up-to-date knowledge about sexually transmitted infections, family planning methods and those specialist services, referral agencies and resources which can be utilized. Individuals will require specialist training to advance this work. There should also be consistent lines of good support which are built into the ethos of the service and firmly placed within the policies and the strategic framework.

Recommendations for future practice

Individual action

This includes the direct contribution that can be made by individual people working in health services and, in particular, within midwifery. Access to good-quality training is essential for all staff, with a regular updating requirement. Such training might cover various facets of sexual health, including aspects of cultural diversity, body image, impact of sexual abuse, HIV infection and prevention, health promotion strategies in collaboration and encouragement of multi-agency contact and involvement. It might also include some personal action planning with some practical ideas for implementing a pro-active role in sexual health promotion. For instance, the standard recording mechanisms such as casenotes and computer records can be used to include specific prompts related to sexual health issues as reminders for staff throughout the pregnancy, labour and delivery, and postnatal period.

Individual and local research is encouraged and the employment of practice based on research evidence. Thus it is important to realize that health promotion and training based on information-giving alone is not effective and needs to be complemented by local action, community initiatives and political motivation.

Local action

Sexual health strategies need to be in place within all midwifery service areas, incorporating those policies and guidelines which may have an impact on services. Management support is essential, with identified lead personnel with responsibility to drive and maintain any agreed level of activity and encourage individual effort.

Activities in clinical/hospital areas and during care in the community might include overt displays of leaflets in a range of service areas, posters advertising the midwifery interest and involvement with sexual health, and inclusion of information about sexual health with first booking letter. Many women are offered HIV counselling and testing at booking, which provides a good opportunity for discussion. An integral space devoted to sexual health on women's record notes, for use at booking, during pre- and postnatal care and when being discharged to the care of the primary care team is a useful reminder to staff.

Close collaboration between health professionals and others involved with service delivery is urged. Involvement with a wide range of external agencies is recommended, both at a local and national level, to encourage good communication and collaboration towards improved care and service delivery. Many services have already been active in establishing maternity liaison groups which can include a range of members to represent local sexual health concerns.

Monitoring, evaluation and review systems which include a user perspective are important so that there is good evidence of work being achieved and a regular opportunity to review practice. This can also be incorporated into the mechanism for informing the purchasing/ commissioning authorities and funding bodies about any contractual concerns. Provision of clear evidence of a need for training in a specific area of work can be a persuasive tool for arguing for supportive funding.

Community action

Community involvement is an area where services can become sensitive to the needs of the local population and particular target areas can be prioritized. It might include the following.

- Greater collaboration with community groups, voluntary agencies and schools through local education authorities, higher profile activities with local press and media and increased involvement with general practice services and other primary care workers. Again emphasis on research-based practice is encouraged.
- Day release or exchange schemes for midwifery service practitioners can enhance understanding and acquaint individuals with key local services like community-based family planning clinics, genito-urinary medicine services, statutory and voluntary drug agencies and others.
- Multi-agency work can be undertaken by and with other services, community leaders and individuals to establish practical methods of raising the profile of sexual health promotion and HIV prevention and encouraging greater sensitivity to local needs.

Political action

Increased support for broad-based sexual health promotion activity by national midwifery and nursing organizational bodies is urged. The importance of having political support at a national and local government level should not be underestimated. Where such support is available it is evident that creative effort can achieve results. An example of this is seen in the establishment of needle exchange schemes, and increased sexual health services for young people in response to targets set in *The health of the nation* report (Department of Health, 1992). Adequate funding is essential for establishing greater numbers of comprehensive sexual health promotion initiatives within all areas of midwifery service delivery, including all those statutory and non-statutory external agencies who could offer support.

Summary of key points

- Midwives are well-placed to play an active and creative role in the field of sexual health promotion. There is encouragement to do so by the professional organizations and by government guidelines.
- Midwives need support to play a positive role in sexual health promotion. This may include maintaining access to current information, establishing good communication networks with local specialist services, identifying individual and service specific training, and emphasizing sexual health promotion within the service contracts.
- A good understanding of the various models and theories of health promotion should enable the practitioner and those managing the service to consider using a broad range of approaches within the individual's working practice and formally integrating these into the policy and structures of the organization. These need to be sensitive to the particular needs of the surrounding community and responsive to the cultural diversities.
- It is recognized that the dimensions of sexual health promotion are enormous, that some important issues have not been dealt with and some aspects have only been mentioned briefly. Further in-depth discussion can be found in the References and Further reading.

References

Ades, A., Davison, C., Holland, F. *et al.* 1993: Vertically transmitted HIV infection in the British Isles. *British Medical Journal* 306, 1296–9.

Aggleton, P. 1992: Models of HIV/AIDS health promotion. In Jones, P. (ed.), *HIV prevention: a working guide for professionals*. London: Health Education Authority.

Aggleton, P. and Homans, H. (ed.) 1988: *Social aspects of AIDS*. East Sussex: The Falmer Press.

Armstrong, E. and Gordon, P. 1992: *Sexualities*. London: Family Planning Association.

Collins 1992: *Softback English dictionary*. Glasgow: Harper Collins.

Department of Health 1992: *The health of the nation: a strategy for health in England*. London: HMSO.

Department of Health 1993a: *Targeting practice: the contribution of nurses, midwives and health visitors*. London: HMSO.

Department of Health 1993b: *Changing childbirth: report of the expert maternity group*. London: HMSO.

Department of Health 1995a: *Making it happen: public health – the contribution, role and development of nurses, midwives and health visitors*. London: SNMAC.

Department of Health 1995b: *HIV and AIDS health promotion: an evolving strategy.* G2/001 3484 1P 8k Nov 95 (21). London: DOH.

Downie, R.S., Tannahill, C. and Tannahill, A. 1996: *Health promotion: models and values.* Oxford: Oxford University Press.

Doyal, L., Naidoo, J. and Wilton, T. (eds) 1994: *AIDS: setting a feminist agenda.* London: Taylor and Francis.

ENB (English National Board for Nursing, Midwifery and Health Visiting) 1994: *Sexual health education and training: guidelines for good practice in the teaching of nurses, midwives and health visitors.* London: ENB.

Ewles, L. and Simnett, I. 1995: *Promoting health: a practical guide.* London: Scutari Press.

Health Education Authority 1994: *Health update 4: sexual health.* London: Health Education Authority.

Holland, J., Ramazanoglu, C., Scott, S. and Thomson, R. 1994: Desire, risk and control: the body as a site of contestation. In Doyal, L., Naidoo, J. and Wilton, T. (eds), *AIDS: setting a feminist agenda.* London: Taylor and Francis, 61–79.

IPPF (International Planned Parenthood Federation) 1994: *Sexual health.* IPPF Statement 4. London: IPPF.

Kabukaba, J.J. and Young, P. 1992: Midwifery and body fluid contamination. *British Medical Journal* 305, 226.

Llewellyn-Jones, D. 1990: *Sexually transmitted diseases.* London: Faber and Faber.

McNab, M. 1993: Ventures in wonderland: HIV prevention and women's perspectives of collaboration. Unpublished masters dissertation.

Naidoo, J. and Wills, J. 1994: *Health promotion: foundations for practice.* London: Baillière Tindall.

Panos 1990: *Triple jeopardy – women and AIDS.* London: The Panos Institute.

Public Health Laboratory Service AIDS Centre, Communicable Disease Surveillance & Scottish Centre for Infection & Environmental Health 1996: AIDS & HIV quarterly surveillance tables. *Communicable Diseases Report* 10(32).

Rawson, D. 1992: The growth of health promotion theory and its rational reconstruction. In Bunton, R. and MacDonald, G. (eds), *Health promotion: disciplines and diversity.* London: Kings Fund.

RCN (Royal College of Nursing) 1995: *Challenging the present, improving the future.* London: RCN.

Richardson, D. 1987: *Women and the AIDS crisis.* London: Pandora Press.

Sharp, C., Maychell, K. and Walton, I. 1993: Issues, information and teaching materials on HIV and AIDS for nurses: a research study. Nursing and AIDS: Material Matters. Slough: National Foundation for Educational Research (NFER).

Szarewski, A. and Guillebaud, J. 1994: *Contraception: a users handbook.* Oxford: Oxford University Press.

Thomas, B.G. 1996: Teenage sexual health promotion. *Journal of the Institute of Health Education.* 34(3), 89–94.

Tones, K., Tilford, S. and Robinson, Y. 1990: *Health education: effectiveness and efficiency.* London: Chapman and Hall.

UKCC (United Kingdom Central Council for Nursing, Midwifery and Health Visiting) 1994: AIDS and HIV infection. *UKCC Registrar's Letter.* CJR/RHP/CS9. London: UKCC.

Wellings, K., Field, J., Johnson, A. and Wadsworth, J. 1994: *Sexual behaviour in Britain*. London: Penguin.

Willy, M., Dhillon, G., Loewen, N., Wesley, R. and Henderson, D. 1990: Adverse exposures and universal precautions practices among a group of highly exposed health professionals. *Infection Control and Hospital Epidemiology* 11(7), 351–6.

Wilton, T. 1994: Feminism and the erotics of health promotion. In Doyal, L., Naidoo, J. and Wilton, T. (eds), *AIDS: setting a feminist agenda*. London: Taylor & Francis, 80–94.

WHO (World Health Organization) 1986a: *Concepts for sexual health*. EUR/ICP/MCP 521. Copenhagen: WHO.

WHO 1986b: *Ottawa Charter for health promotion*. Ontario: World Health Organization & Health and Welfare.

Further reading

Bowler, I. 1993: They're not the same as us: midwives' stereotypes of South Asian descent maternity patients. *Sociology of Health & Illness* 15(2), 157–78.

Devane, D. 1996: Sexuality and midwifery. *British Journal of Midwifery* 4(8), 413–19.

ENB (English National Board for Nursing, Midwifery and Health Visiting) 1994: *Sexual health education and training: guidelines for good practice in the teaching of nurses, midwives and health visitors*. London: ENB.

RCN (Royal College of Nursing) 1996: HIV & AIDS position paper no. 16.

Robinson, J. 1996: The SEX model of sexual health. *British Journal of Midwifery* 4(8), 420–4.

Wellings, K., Field, J., Johnson, A. and Wadsworth, J. 1994: *Sexual behaviour in Britain*. London: Penguin.

14

Promoting breastfeeding

Lea Jamieson and Louise M. Long

Promoting the health of newborn babies by supporting breastfeeding has long been the responsibility of midwives. It has now been established without doubt that physiologically breast milk is the ideal food for human babies. Minchin (1989) and Lawrence (1994) detail most of the current evidence and compare modified cow's milk with human milk, showing the former's inadequacies and the ultimate effects on health. A sociological perspective is required by both mother and midwife. This chapter identifies the position of the professional in relation to breastfeeding outcomes. It identifies the research which can be used to both inform and develop a midwife as a skilful breastfeeding supporter. A health promotion process is explored to enable the practitioner to examine their own practice and develop their skills in the teaching and promotion of breastfeeding. The focus of using research to guide both health promotion and the developing skill is maintained throughout.

Exploring the midwife's and woman's perspective on promoting breastfeeding

So what is actually needed when promoting breastfeeding? How may the number of babies receiving breast milk be increased? The answers to these questions are complex and involve many factors. At first it may appear as simple as encouraging more women to breastfeed their babies. To this end many posters advertising that 'breast is best' have been designed and have formed the centre of health promotion campaign efforts. However examination of the current situation and trends in breastfeeding reveals more appropriate answers to these questions and identifies quite a different educational need.

As stated in Chapter 1, a 'need' occurs when a set of circumstances requires a course of action. The *Changing childbirth* report (Department of Health, 1993) sought to assess the circumstances in general terms within maternity services. It established the 'felt need' (what women say they want from the service), responded to the 'expressed need', by producing guidelines on how the service may be run, and encouraged 'comparative need' (the assessing of gaps and inequality of provision). It placed the 'women as the centre' of service provision and all aspects of this care, and it sets out that all women need information to make an informed choice about all aspects of their care. It is within this context that breastfeeding promotion must be placed.

The particular set of circumstances that prevail nationally with breast-feeding can be derived from the findings of the most recent in a series of four *Infant feeding* reports (White *et al.*, 1992) conducted by the Social Survey Division of the then Office of Population Censuses and Surveys (OPCS). This is the largest, most comprehensive report into infant feeding in the UK. In tackling 'need' the local situation also bears investigation. The OPCS study shows us the characteristics of women who breastfeed and how successful these women then are when they start. This is helpful in ascertaining where breastfeeding promotion should be targeted.

The characteristics of women who start breastfeeding

White *et al.* (1992) report that the 'classic' breastfeeding mother:

- is having her first baby,
- is aged 30 or over,
- was a non-smoker before pregnancy,
- has a partner,
- is from social class 1 or 2,
- has been breastfed herself, and
- lives in the south of England.

They also conclude that the decision to breastfeed can be made as early as school years and that later it is greatly influenced by peer group.

Educational level is also a factor. The woman having her first baby who left full-time education after the age of 19 is more likely to breastfeed than the woman who left school aged 16 or under. Theses factors have often contributed to stereotyping these women into the 'NCT (National Child-birth Trust) type' (Green *et al.*, 1990). This 'type' is highly motivated, avails herself of information and preparation, and usually has a clear idea of what she wants.

The percentage of women who initially start to breastfeed varies depending on geographical area and there appears to be a 'north/south' divide in this respect. The further north one travels throughout England and into Scotland, the less and less breastfeeding is seen, health care professionals become less developed in their skill and therefore those women who do start have even less chance of skilled professional help.

What happens to the women who start breastfeeding?

These facts are probably the most important when considering breastfeeding promotion. Do all women who start breastfeeding continue until they have breastfed for as long as they intended to? Does being the motivated 'NCT type' (Green *et al.*, 1990) ensure success?

White *et al.* (1992) report that of the national average 65 per cent of women who start breastfeeding after the birth of their baby, 12 per cent have encountered a difficulty in trying to establish the process and, because of this, have given up by the time they leave hospital. Altogether, by the end of the second week, 20 per cent of those who have started have given up. The further 8 per cent who make up this figure, have given up after discharge from hospital. This means that during the time when midwifery help is at its most accessible, the steepest decline in breastfeeding is seen. This fact is key when considering how breastfeeding rates may be increased. It also shows that the time spent in hospital is the most significant with established breastfeeding.

The most common reason cited by mothers for discontinuing breastfeeding during the first week is sore nipples or breasts. Other reasons are insufficient milk, the baby wouldn't suck, and breastfeeding took too long/was tiring. None of the mothers at this stage have given up because they had breastfed for as long as they had intended to, indeed this only becomes cited as a reason with mothers who have given up at 3 months or later.

As stated, these are national average figures. There are local variations. The national figures help to focus attention on the contribution a local area might be making.

All the reasons given by mothers as to why they have given up can be attributed to incorrectly attaching the baby to the breast. Indeed this is the trigger for most other problems occurring and the eventual discontinuing of breastfeeding by the mother. Figure 14.1 sets out the cascade of unsuccessful breastfeeding diagrammatically. Unless the professional has the knowledge and skill to help the mother, failure to establish breastfeeding becomes more likely with all the emotional consequences this involves (Wilby, 1995).

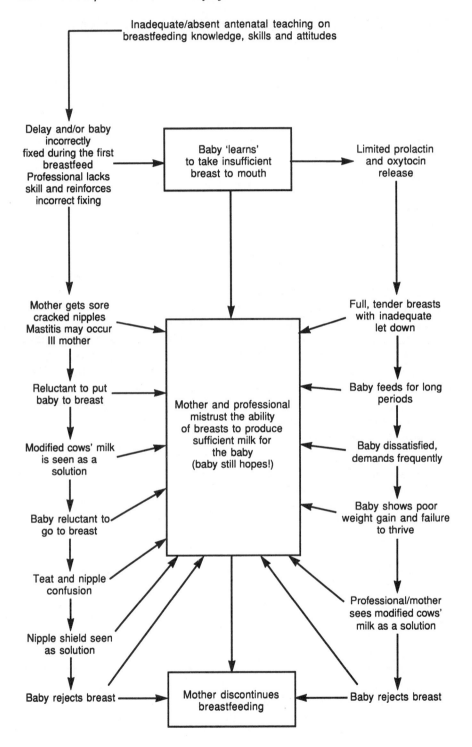

Figure 14.1 Cascade of unsuccessful breastfeeding

Healthcare professionals' support of women who want to breastfeed

The key or lead professional who is with the mother during pregnancy, birth and during the postnatal period is the midwife. Initially she supports the mother by giving information about breastfeeding. Later she uses her skills to teach the mother how to attach the baby correctly to the breast. Encouragement given with the additional skills builds confidence in the mother and this completes the midwife's role.

Unfortunately, training for midwives in this role varies in quality and is haphazard in process. The necessary knowledge is not always imparted and this may lead to the giving of information in a way that makes informed choice impossible. The practical skill of teaching a mother correct attachment is rarely taught. All too often the education received covers knowledge-based lectures on the physiology of lactation or the constituents of breast milk, etc. How this is related to practice is then dependent on the adequacy of the clinical placement and the quality of the role-model provided by the qualified midwife seen by the student. The student picks up skills on an apprenticeship basis seeing other qualified midwives at work. The shortfalls of learning breastfeeding support skills in this way are clear.

The student midwife is at risk of learning effective, research-based approaches with inadequate application to practice. She may not even notice the mismatch between her newly learnt knowledge and the practice observed. A good example of this is advice to 'rest' sore nipples. This may appear to the student to be a logical step in the circumstances, something which she will adopt into her own practice. In fact what is needed is for the mother and baby to be shown correct attachment which is pain free causing no trauma to the nipple. This essentially requires specific application of physiology and skill on the part of the practitioner.

The results of this haphazard skill-acquiring are highlighted by the frequent complaints from mothers of inconsistent and conflicting advice. The damage this causes to successfully establishing breastfeeding and to the credibility of the professionals cannot be overestimated. The newly delivered mother, who may have had no preparation for breastfeeding, who is tired and vulnerable after a long labour, becomes totally dependent on the quality of knowledge and skill of the midwife who happens to be on duty. Whether she now starts going down the 'cascade of unsuccessful breastfeeding' and how far she gets becomes a lottery. If, at the first feed, she meets a skilled practitioner who enables correct fixing and she can subsequently reproduce this she will be well on the road to fulfilling her choice to breastfeed. If, however, the first feed is delayed and/or the practitioner lacks skill, the cascade of unsuccessful feeding may have been triggered. Now the mother is dependent on encountering a midwife with ever increasing skill as she moves further and further down the cascade. Clearly, any midwife offering care at the last point on the cascade will need much greater skill than a midwife offering support earlier. The skill is to reverse the loss of confidence in the mother and the confusion and poor habits learned by the baby. Effective promotion of breastfeeding with adequate skills cuts across the cascade and prevents a negative outcome (Fig. 14.2).

Achieving the skilled practitioner

Midwifery education has undergone many changes over the past few years but the rules related to outcome (rule 33) remain open to inter-pretation regarding level and content of breastfeeding skills and knowl-edge. UNICEF (1994) recommended at least 18 hours of breastfeeding training for health care staff supporting mothers. The UKCC Post-registration and Practice (PREP) legislation came into effect in April 1995. Under this legislation midwives are required to continue professional development with areas of study immediately relevant to practice (UKCC, 1994). It is hoped that this, along with midwifery education moving into higher education, will provide opportunities for develop-ing and offering breastfeeding courses in the form of modules. One such module is described by Dykes (1995) at the University of Central Lancashire. These courses, along with in-service training packages, go some way at least to improving the situation.

Policies and attitudes to breastfeeding

Sometimes a breastfeeding policy is seen as an answer, at least in part, to this problem. It attempts to provide standardized advice and govern what happens in practice. Unfortunately these policies and their implementa-tion in practice are often found to be inadequate. Garforth and Garcia (1989) conducted a national survey of breastfeeding policies produced by maternity units and found huge variations and anomalies within policies. These were not consistent with available research and may in some cases actively hinder the establishment of successful feeding. In their discussion Garforth and Garcia acknowledge that attitudes to breastfeeding vary tremendously. They state that there are midwives who

> saw initiating breastfeeding and supporting the woman in breastfeeding as 'the stuff of midwifery', an important skill they had to offer and worthy of time and effort. Conversely there were others who saw it as an optional extra to be tacked on at the end of routines (such as examining and weighing the baby . . . etc) if there was time before the room was needed for someone else. Occasionally breastfeeding was omitted by default.

The differing attitudes and priorities of midwives are surrounded by the wider context of culture and experiences and each woman's individ-ual view of their own bodies (Raphael-Leff, 1990). Advertising of infant

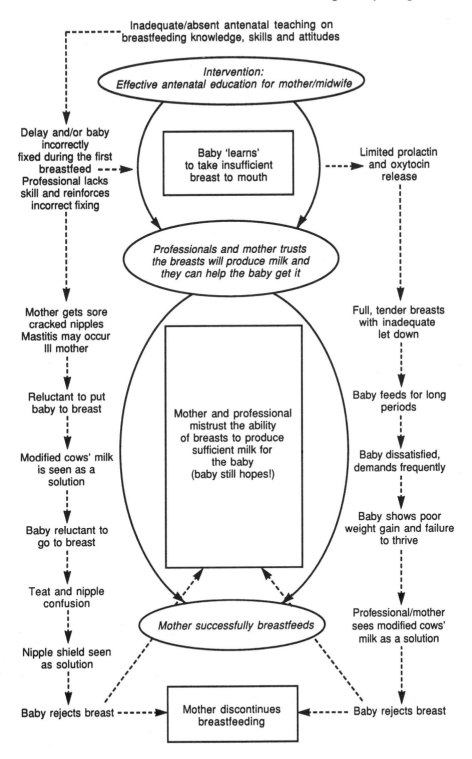

Figure 14.2 Cascade of unsuccessful breastfeeding with intervention

formula (Palmer, 1988), our own immediate culture (Maher, 1992), gender issues (Aston and Bates, 1996), and how we were fed as babies are all said to play a part in whether we decide to breastfeed, how motivated we are to continue and how we help a mother to breastfeed. Any breastfeeding promotion and education must encompass examination of all these aspects.

In their discussion, Garforth and Garcia (1989) also address the issue of inconsistent and conflicting advice. They suggest 'intensive in-service' training is needed to inform and update all levels of staff on evidence-based practice and decision-making skills. They also comment that the hospital environment must also be conducive to implementing indi-vidualized care with flexible 'routines' such as mealtimes that encourage 'baby-led' feeding. Managers need to work closely with midwifery educa-tionalists so that any in-service training undertaken can be transferred into the clinical practice setting more effectively. The intervention described later in this chapter responds to such recommendations. As midwifery training and education move into higher education these issues will be and are being addressed for tomorrow's practitioners and in part for today's.

The conclusions which can be drawn from this analysis of current circumstances and hence the 'need' for breastfeeding promotion are two-fold. They involve mothers and midwives and can be summarized as follows:

- All mothers need information on breastfeeding in order to make an informed choice. Mothers who are ambivalent or who have decided to breastfeed need sensitive, appropriate, realistic preparation during the antenatal period to give them confidence and autonomy for breast-feeding. They need an opportunity to reflect on their own attitudes, how they were fed as babies and what the 'norm' is within their peer group. They need knowledge of how their breasts work to produce milk so that they understand how breastfeeding becomes established. And lastly they need to have practised the skill of how to position their baby correctly at the breast and recognize this has occurred from the very first feed, thus preventing the start of the unsuccessful breastfeeding cascade.
- Midwives need to examine their attitudes and to determine where they, as individuals, fall on the motivation line of helping a mother breastfeed her baby. They need to acknowledge whether they would breastfeed or have breastfed their own baby and the influence of that experience. They also need to make sure that their knowledge is up to date. Knowledge about breastfeeding may have changed considerably since their own initial training or refresher course. Then they need to be taught a systematic approach (the skill) to helping a mother to help herself (Long, 1995; Jamieson, 1995) to attach her baby correctly.

'Getting it Together' – Breastfeeding Workshops

To address the needs identified in current research the 'Getting it Together' Breastfeeding Workshop educational package was developed and first run at a maternity unit in London in 1990. It included the three identified areas of knowledge, skill and attitudes and a cyclical educational approach was used to develop and evaluate the package. This approach is illustrated in Fig. 14.3 and could be used to explore answers to other health promotional problems. Sometimes just writing down what is happening clinically adds clarity to the real 'problem'. In terms of breastfeeding it was found that there was need for a consistent step-by-step approach. The approach was developed, implemented and then evaluated. At this point either the problem is solved or partially solved and a new 'need' has emerged and the cycle begins again. The Breastfeeding Workshops worked well and indicated a further need for health visitors to have a 'sustaining breastfeeding workshop' and so the cycle repeated.

Aims of the Breastfeeding Workshop

Evaluation can only be achieved when the goals of an educational experience are clearly stated. Breastfeeding Workshop day aims were as follows:

- To acknowledge the skill and expertise of the midwives and present the Workshop as something which builds and enhances the experienced practitioner.
- To ensure that a high level of accurate knowledge is held by the midwives teaching mothers.
- To teach midwives an approach which gives autonomy to mothers both within the learning experience and to use later in their real-life experience.
- To express the skill of attaching the baby in clear steps which can be easily understood and transferred to the mothers.
- To guide the midwives in providing an educational environment in which the individual mother identifies, explores and satisfies her need for knowledge and skill specific to her ultimate success in breastfeeding.
- To offer opportunity to discuss and observe newly delivered mothers' skills and observations within the breastfeeding process.
- To identify attitudes within breastfeeding that enhance success, reflect on these and encourage them in the educational exchange.

The Workshop day can be expressed as a flowchart (Fig. 14.4) and it can be seen how the aims are addressed for the different participants.

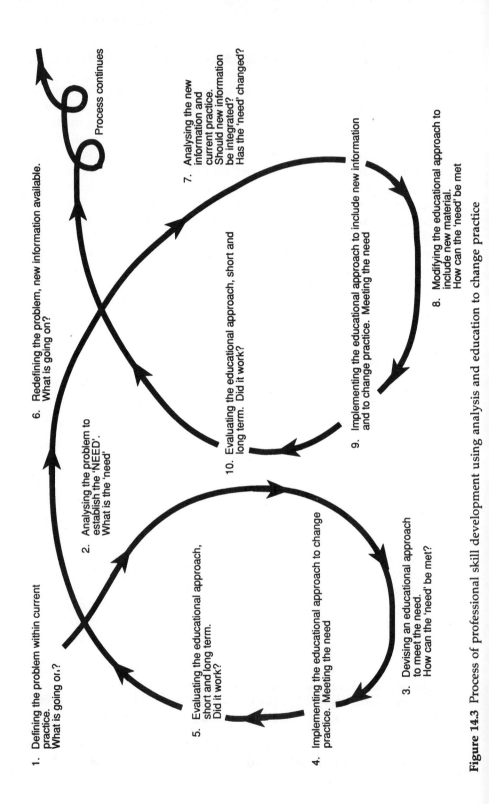

1. Defining the problem within current practice.
   What is going on.?

2. Analysing the problem to establish the 'NEED'.
   What is the 'need'

3. Devising an educational approach to meet the need.
   How can the 'need' be met?

4. Implementing the educational approach to change practice. Meeting the need

5. Evaluating the educational approach, short and long term.
   Did it work?

6. Redefining the problem, new information available.
   What is going on?

7. Analysing the new information and current practice.
   Should new information be integrated?
   Has the 'need' changed?

8. Modifying the educational approach to include new material.
   How can the 'need' be met

9. Implementing the educational approach to include new information and to change practice. Meeting the need

10. Evaluating the educational approach, short and long term. Did it work?

Process continues

Figure 14.3 Process of professional skill development using analysis and education to change practice

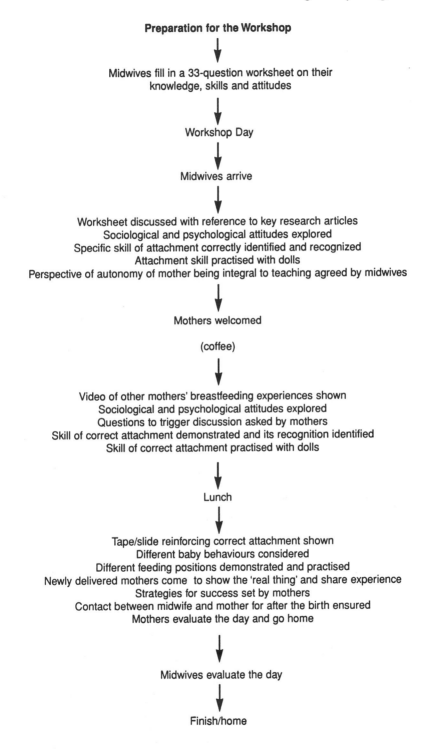

Figure 14.4 Flowchart of 'Getting it Together' Breastfeeding Workshop day (Modified from Jamieson, 1990).

Clarity of focus

All education material should clearly address the needs of the midwife and cover the application of their knowledge, skills and attitudes. The three examples from the Breastfeeding Workshop worksheet show how this can be achieved.

Knowledge

- How effective is a humilactor in raising prolactin levels? Can you support your answer?
- How would you use this knowledge when helping a mother to express her milk for a baby in a neonatal unit/nursery?

Skills

- What is the first question you ask yourself if it appears that the baby is not obtaining sufficient milk?
- Describe briefly what you would do in order to answer your first question.

Attitudes

- How easy is it to work and continue breastfeeding? Place your cross on the line.
  Very easy _____ Impossible
- Consider why you put your cross just where you did. Consider how your personal view could influence the advice you give a mother.
- If you could only give a mother who wants to return to work and breastfeed three principles to follow, what would they be?

The result of exploring the questions is that the baseline knowledge of the midwife increases alongside confidence. At the start of the Workshop day the discussion focuses on the evidence that informs the answers.

Focus on mothers

Mothers start with a welcome by their midwives with coffee, and watch a video of mothers talking about their experiences. Teaching in small groups (one midwife to two mothers) enables individually tailored responses, ensuring each mother acquires the knowledge and skills she needs within her family circumstances.

Lunch is shared and followed by a large group session where the skill is reinforced both by interactive demonstration and a tape slide. A mother who has attended a workshop comes to share her 'real' experience and a correctly attached baby can be observed. Different feeding positions are practised. A mother having twins or anticipating a Caesarean section discusses her specific needs at this time and practises positions to help her. The facilitator intervenes, suggests, discusses and encourages the midwife according to her individual level of skill.

Contact for the postnatal period between the mother and the midwife is arranged and finally the mothers evaluate the day and leave. The day ends with the midwives reflecting on all parts of the day, observing and reporting on their own learning.

The steps for correct fixing (Fig. 14.5)

These are taught first to the midwives and then by the midwives to the mothers. It is important to use simple clear instructions that can be repeated and remembered. It is vital the mother understands the rationale behind the detail of the steps she is learning.

Having taught these steps, the facilitator confirms that both mothers and midwives can demonstrate their learning and evaluates the day with first the mothers and then the midwives.

Identifying a problem and analysing it to demonstrate a precise need leads to a focused intervention which can be tested for effectiveness. The process can be applied to a small or large problem. The effect of the intervention is to prevent the discontinuation at any point in the cascade, but ideally antenatally (*see* Fig. 14.2).

Evaluation of the Breastfeeding Workshop

The educational teaching Breastfeeding Workshop package was first run at a maternity unit in London in 1990. Both long-term and short-term evaluation accompanied the programme as it was started. The evaluation process had four aims:

1. To highlight any differences in confidence between the control group (see later) and the Workshop attendees group.
2. To assess the number of mothers in each group who were still breastfeeding between 8 and 21 weeks postnatally.
3. To assess any changes in the midwives' knowledge and practice after attending the Workshop.
4. To assess to what extent the day had been enjoyable, non-threatening and a learning experience for midwives and mothers.

In summary, both the qualitative and quantitative findings showed that the Breastfeeding Workshops were successful at meeting their objectives.

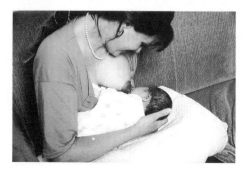

Step one. Hold your baby horizontal at the level of your breasts facing inwards. This position gives the baby the optimum conditions.

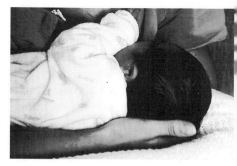

Step two. Support your baby's head by making your hand a shelf under her ear (your wrist should be approximately at the baby's neck). This gives the baby the freedom to extend her neck and position comfortably on the breast. The baby is not in any way forced on to the breast.

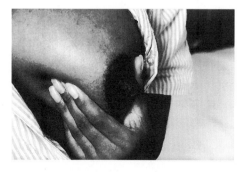

Step three. Make your breast a shape that fits the baby's open mouth by making a V underneath the breast with your hand. Do not lift the breast; hold it at its resting position so that it does not drop when your hand is removed.

Step four. When the baby opens her mouth wide, bring her towards the breast aiming her nose to the nipple tip. Take care to get a large part of the breast well over the bottom jaw of the baby. To avoid soreness, the most important part of the breast to get into the baby's mouth is the part of the areola next to the bottom jaw. Always bring the baby to the breast to achieve a comfortable final position, as leaning forward causes backache.

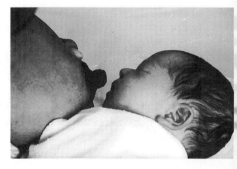

Figure 14.5 The steps for correct attachment

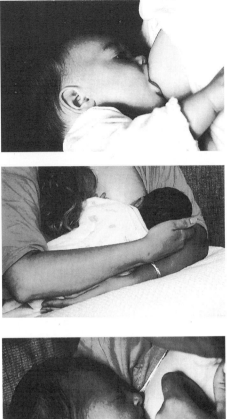

Step five. Check for signs of correct attachment: no pain, rhythmic sucking with pauses, chin pressed against the breast, and a small movement in front of the ear indicating swallowing.

Step six. When the signs of correct attachment are present, if you feel confident and comfortable, gently let go of your breast and bring your hand round to the nappy so the baby is cradled in your arm with her head nestled at your elbow. Relax your shoulders down if they have risen up and lean back into the chair or pillows. It is possible to use your other hand to stroke your baby or have a drink!

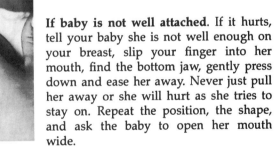

If baby is not well attached. If it hurts, tell your baby she is not well enough on your breast, slip your finger into her mouth, find the bottom jaw, gently press down and ease her away. Never just pull her away or she will hurt as she tries to stay on. Repeat the position, the shape, and ask the baby to open her mouth wide.

Long-term evaluation (from Clifton and Long, 1990)

A long-term (up to 12 weeks postnatal) follow-up study was devised to ascertain the effects of the Workshop on mothers who attended, particularly where success with breastfeeding was concerned and on midwives' knowledge and practice. It involved both qualitative and quantitative perspectives using self-report. Questionnaires and semi-structured interviews were used to obtain the information. The evaluation process can be seen in Fig. 14.6.

Long-term evaluation of mothers

The first group of mothers recruited formed a 'control' group. This group were collected before the Breastfeeding Workshop programme began and

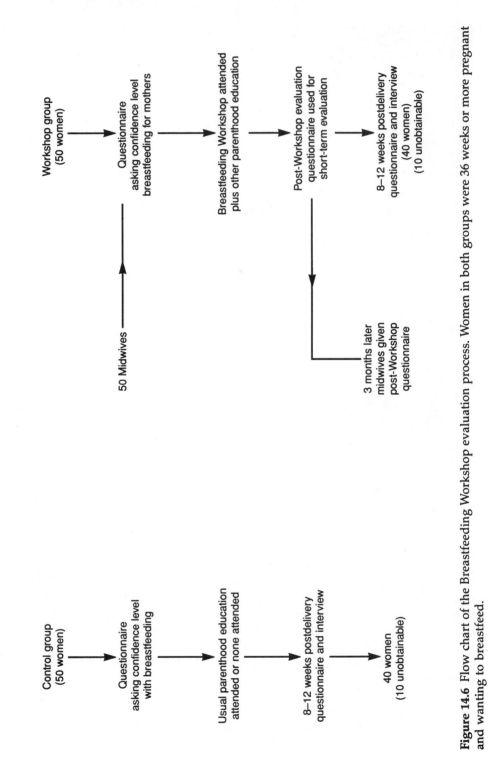

Figure 14.6 Flow chart of the Breastfeeding Workshop evaluation process. Women in both groups were 36 weeks or more pregnant and wanting to breastfeed.

were later compared with the Workshop attendee group. There were fifty mothers in this group. All of them were at least 36 weeks pregnant and definitely wanted to breastfeed. They were recruited from the hospital and a community-based antenatal clinic waiting room by being approached by the researchers. To collect this group of women, all women who were 36 weeks pregnant were approached. The first fifty who met the criteria were then included after their consent was obtained.

The second group of mothers were the Workshop attendees group. They too were at least 36 weeks pregnant and wanted to breastfeed. These women had responded to the advertising of the Workshops in the antenatal clinic and obviously decided to attend. They were recruited just before the beginning of the Workshop day by the researchers until we had fifty women.

Both groups of women were given a questionnaire which asked how confident they were about their decision to breastfeed. The categories they were asked to tick were: not at all confident; uncertain; quite confident; and very confident. Demographic details were collected for all women regarding age, parity, ethnic group, occupation, if with a partner, parentcraft attended, and expected date of delivery.

The different groups then either attended the Workshop, had traditional antenatal classes or both or neither. Information about when the women gave birth was collected by the researchers from the hospital birth register. These were then matched with the expected date of delivery and any babies that were born before 38 weeks gestation or who weighed above the 90th centile or below the 10th centile were excluded.

Appointments were then made with the women for one of the researchers to visit them at home to complete a follow-up questionnaire and have an interview at between 8 and 12 weeks postnatally.

At the follow-up interview the mothers were asked how they were now feeding their babies and about their breastfeeding experience, however long or short this had been. They answered questions about their confidence, whether they had any problems and, if they were in the Workshop group, whether they thought the Workshop had helped them prepare for breastfeeding and whether they would recommend the Workshop to other mothers.

Long-term evaluation of midwives

The long-term evaluation process with the midwives started with a pre-Workshop questionnaire. This was to establish some idea of the knowledge level amongst the midwives in the unit. It gave ten factors and asked the midwives to select the three that were the most important with *establishing* and *continuing* breastfeeding. The list was as follows:

- Attitude of mother
- Good supply of milk

- Mother's general health
- Mother's family/social history
- Nipple size and shape
- Positioning of infant
- Support by husband or partner
- Skilled health visiting support
- Skilled midwifery support
- Type of delivery

The other question they were asked was, on a scale of 1–5, how confident they felt with supporting a mother to breastfeed (1 was not at all confident and 5 was totally confident). The follow-up at approximately 3 months involved them completing a questionnaire which asked whether they had more knowledge about breastfeeding as a result of the Workshop, how successful they were with using the approach taught, whether they noticed any differences with mothers who had attended a Workshop in clinical practice postnatally and whether they would recommend the Workshop to other midwives.

Findings involving the mothers

Forty mothers were followed up in each group. Ten women from each group were either excluded due to their baby being born before 38 weeks gestation or its weight being above or below the 90th or 10th centile. Some mothers had moved house and were no longer contactable.

The two groups were then compared in terms of age, parity, which parenthood classes they had attended (other than the Workshop if they were in the Workshop group), their occupation, ethnic group, if they had a partner and type of delivery they had had. Comparison of the groups did not reveal any significant differences other than with parity and the other parenthood education (Table 14.1).

It is perhaps surprising that the majority of the Workshop attendees group (who had selected themselves) were primiparous women. Parenthood education is often more attractive to women who are expecting their first baby and hence they often attend in greater numbers. Because of this difference and the variety of parenthood education attended (Table 14.2) quantitative comparison between the two groups was considered impossible to interpret in a meaningful way. In retrospect it would have made

Table 14.1 Parity of the mothers involved in long-term evaluation

Parity	Workshop attendees	Control group
0	90% (36)	52% (21)
> 0	10% (4)	47% (19)

Table 14.2 Parenthood education attended by the mothers involved in long-term evaluation

	Workshop attendees	*Control group*
Hospital classes	75.5% (29)	55% (22)
National Childbirth Trust (NCT)	2.5% (1)	2.5% (1)
Active Birth	12.5% (5)	2.5% (1)
Hospital classes and NCT	7.5% (3)	0
None	5% (2)	40% (16)

for easier comparison if all women from both groups had been primiparas and this should probably have been anticipated at the beginning of the project.

Because of these differences, it was also impossible to interpret the data obtained about confidence. The Workshop group showed higher levels of confidence both before and after the Workshop than the control group, but we cannot forward any conclusions about these findings.

When it came to the question of how many mothers were still breast-feeding at between 8 and 12 weeks, the Workshop group showed higher numbers (Table 14.3). These results showed that there were 20 per cent more mothers in the Workshop group still breastfeeding at between 8 and 12 weeks.

The qualitative information from the mothers was overwhelmingly positive. All women (100 per cent) said that the Workshop had helped them and that they would recommend it to other mothers. Thirty-five per cent of the Workshop group said that they had developed some soreness during the first few days. All of those mothers said they realized this was due to incorrect attachment and were able to correct this as the baby and they got better at attachment. Most obviously overcame this problem.

The mothers who had attended a Workshop but were bottlefeeding at the 8–12 week interview were interesting. Two had had uterine infections which had resulted in re-admission to hospital and them discontinuing breastfeeding. Two women had never really achieved correct attachment and two had discontinued due to family/partner pressure.

Table 14.3 Method of feeding used between 8 and 12 weeks by the mothers involved in long-term evaluation

	Workshop attendees	*Control group*
Breast	75% (30)	55% (22)
Bottle	15% (6)	35% (14)
Mixed	10% (4)	10% (4)

Table 14.4 Results of the pre-Workshop
questionnaire for midwives: levels of
confidence in helping mothers to breastfeed

Level 1 (not at all confident)	0
Level 2	0
Level 3	24.5% (13)
Level 4	42.5% (22)
Level 5 (totally confident)	33.9% (18)

Findings involving the midwives

The first part of the evaluation was the pre-Workshop questionnaire.
There were fifty-three midwives in the group on which we based these
pre-Workshop results. First we asked how confident they felt about
helping mothers to breastfeed. The scale was from 1 to 5 (1 = not at
all confident and 5 = totally confident). The results (Table 14.4) showed
that whilst confidence levels were high, few midwives felt totally confident.

The result of the pre-Workshop questionnaire section that asked the
midwives to choose the three factors most likely to help with establishing
and continuing breastfeeding (out of a list of ten) were as follows:

- The most popular combination, chosen by 35.8 per cent (19) of the
  midwives, was:
  - Attitude of mother
  - Positioning of infant
  - Skilled midwifery support
- The second most popular combination, chosen by 15 per cent (8),
  was:
  - Attitude of mother
  - Positioning of infant
  - Support by husband/partner
- The third most popular combination, chosen by 7.5 per cent (4), was:
  - Attitude of mother
  - Skilled midwifery support
  - Support by husband/partner.

The remaining 41.5 per cent (22) midwives produced very different
combinations. The most unexpected responses were from midwives who
reported the highest level of confidence with helping a mother to
breastfeed!

The follow-up results from the questionnaires involved fifty midwives.
It was carried out approximately 3 months later. Ninety per cent of the
midwives who responded said that they had increased knowledge about
breastfeeding since the Workshop. The second question asked midwives

how successful they had been with using the Workshop approach to correct fixing.

Not successful	0%
Sometimes successful	39.5%
Often successful	27%
Very successful	32%

This showed that all the midwives had had some success with the approach that had been taught.

In answer to the question about being able to recognize women who have attended a Workshop in clinical practice, 90 per cent (45) said yes and 16 per cent (8) said no. Some of the comments that midwives made were:

'I've noticed mothers seem more confident.'
'The mothers who have been to a Workshop are prepared to have a go at fixing themselves'.
'Workshop women need much less help – they seem to know what to do.'
'I end up spending so much time with the women who haven't been – I wish they had!'

All the midwives who had been to a Workshop said they would recommend the Workshop to other midwives.

Conclusion

The conclusions from the results of this study are drawn largely from the qualitative data. Although the women and midwives were all from the same maternity unit and may not be typical of the general midwifery population, the qualitative data collected provides interesting insights into breastfeeding experiences. The fourth aim of the evaluation appeared to have been met in full. All the qualitative information collected was overwhelmingly positive. It is highly significant that all mothers and all midwives would recommend the Workshop to others and made positive comments about it.

The quantitative data are more difficult to assess. Whilst every attempt was made to compare the control and the Workshop groups, the differences of parity and additional parenthood education attended between the two groups remain an obstacle to true comparison.

In view of the parity in particular showing such a large difference, it may have been more helpful to limit the long-term evaluation project to primiparous women only. It was our enthusiasm to include all women which led to these difficulties not being fully realized at the outset.

The question of feeding at 8–12 weeks was one of the most important to the quantitative results. The Workshop group were undoubtedly breast-feeding for longer than the control group. This is despite there being more primiparous women in the Workshop attendees group. Whether this can be put down to attending a Workshop alone is questionable due to sample size. It would be fair to say the trend appears to exist. Qualitative evidence would suggest that the Workshop played a large part. The results certainly compared very favourably with the OPCS study (White *et al.*, 1992) and with the national figures on prevalence of breastfeeding between 8 and 12 weeks postnatally.

We concluded that most midwives felt quite confident at helping a mother to breastfeed her baby. However this confidence could not be matched when actual knowledge was tested. Slightly less than half the midwives were up-to-date enough to identify the correct combination of factors from the research-based list presented. This showed a real need for education. Although knowledge was not tested again at 3 months, the vast majority of midwives did report greater knowledge post-Workshop. Hence we can conclude that the Workshop had achieved its educational function.

The majority of midwives could recognize mothers who had attended a Workshop from the level of skill and confidence they had. This adds weight to the education and confidence-boosting function of the Workshop.

The fact that all the midwives who had attended the Workshops would recommend them to other midwives showed overwhelmingly that we had achieved our fourth aim of creating a non-threatening educational environment. This was the most successful qualitative assessment.

Short-term evaluation

Short-term evaluation was carried out at the end of each Workshop. Both mothers and midwives were given the same short questionnaire asking them four questions:

- Have you found the Workshop useful?
- What were the most valuable parts of the day?
- Can you suggest areas for improvement?
- Please add any comments about the Workshop which will help us to decide on the future of this programme.

They were then asked to identify themselves as either a 'pregnant woman', a 'midwife' or 'other'.

Evaluation from all the pregnant women who attended a Workshop was collected until we had 500 completed questionnaires. The findings are as follows:

Responses to the first question: 'Have you found the Workshop useful?

Yes	99.6%	(498)
No	0.4%	(2)
Other/blank	0	

This shows an overwhelmingly positive response to the Workshop. Of the 99.6 per cent who said 'yes', 37.8 per cent (189) qualified 'yes' with other positive words or phrases. Of the two women who said 'no', one woman said, 'I want to bottle-feed' and the other said, 'No, not really' and in both cases the rest of the questionnaire was left blank.

Responses to the second question: 'What were the most valuable parts of the day?'

Practising correct fixing with the dolls	46.6%	(232)
Small group discussion with the midwife and seeing a real mother breastfeeding	43.4%	(217)
The video of mothers talking	5%	(25)
Miscellaneous (see below)	2.6%	(14)
The tape slide presentation summary	2.4%	(12)

Most women actually stated a particular part of the day, although some responded 'all of it; and these were included in the 'miscellaneous' section. It is clear that the small group discussions during which time practising attachment with dolls took place were very successful. If we had been unable to show a real mother breastfeeding, this often came up in the evaluation, suggesting it would have been better to include such a demonstration.

Responses to the third question: 'Can you suggest any areas for improvement?'

No	69%	(345)
Miscellaneous (see below)	21%	(105)
Would have liked more time in discussion groups	5.8%	(29)
Suggested a more up-to-date tape slide was needed	4.2%	(21)

The majority of women (nearly 70 per cent) thought the Workshop worked well. They frequently commented that the mixture of audiovisual aids, discussion and practising with the dolls provided an excellent balance. A new tape slide was produced in response to the evaluation. The suggestions of the miscellaneous group (21 per cent (105)) showed a wide variety of responses, but no single group emerged. A selection of responses are listed below. There were no more than ten women in each group.

- More information about diet.
- The Workshop being too long/too short, too negative/too positive or the parts of the Workshop in a different order.
- To have big group discussion as well as small groups.
- To have more literature available and a suggested book reading list.
- More on the physiological/biological aspects.

Responses to the fourth question: 'Please add any comments which will help us decide the future of this programme'

All responses to this request, where it was answered, were very positive. We divided them into four categories: confidence and knowledge; discussion time with the midwife; being able to ask any questions; and continuing the programme. Some comments from each of the four categories are listed below.

Confidence and knowledge

'Most valuable because it's given me more confidence and made me feel more relaxed.'

'Extremely useful. I didn't have a clue.'

'I think the Workshop is good because it makes you aware of any possible problems and you will hopefully be able to cope with them better.'

Discussion time and the midwife

'I don't think there would have been another opportunity to spend so much time on the subject with such specialised help.'

'Good to have one midwife to so few mothers because you can ask more questions and feel relaxed.'

'Confidence-building and reassuring. I've read everything I could already, but talking with the midwife is most helpful.'

'Wonderful the midwife took time to explain all this.'

Being able to ask any questions

'We were given time to ask what could be seen as daft questions.'

'Nice to be able to ask questions however silly.'

Continuing the programme

'Individual attention as opposed to classes and lectures. The Workshop is great.'

'I think that this is the best time to learn about breastfeeding. Leaving it to the postnatal wards is a bit hectic, so to have this grounding will help in the early days.'

'This sort of Workshop should be encouraged throughout all maternity hospitals.'

Recommendations for midwifery education and practice

Designing the Breastfeeding Workshops has produced an approach that can be applied to any educational need. The most important aspect is not to prejudge an answer but to allow it to evolve in a way that meets needs of both women and midwives. The effectiveness of the package to some extent reflects the time taken to develop it: approximately 10 years. The

Workshops have been used extensively in Tasmania, South Australia where an evaluation of their effectiveness is in progress. In Scotland they have been used to help women in large maternity units and also on a one-to-one basis with community care workers and again there is a project examining outcomes. Most units adopt the Workshop package and lead with midwives, but some centres have taught their local NCT breastfeeding counsellors and others have taught all the midwifery lecturers so that the teaching in the classroom anticipates the needs of women and develops the students' skills from their first contact with pregnant women.

The package created is now being developed to meet the needs of health visitors and it will have the added knowledge, skill and attitudes related to sustaining breastfeeding. A further development is for staff in neonatal units where the approach can be adapted to help the woman wanting to feed a tiny baby. The integral building of confidence in the mother by the professional is important and the trust of the professional in the mother's ability to feed her baby needs to be both present and expressed. Just as in the initiating Breastfeeding Workshops, the information that increases self and body awareness and confidence in their style of mothering is relevant to mothers being helped to sustain feeding or starting to offer their breast for the first time to their preterm baby. The knowledge of the professional for example in relation to the constituents of breast milk is the same for any professional staff helping with breastfeeding.

The recommendations for professional care are to be methodical in approach to both defining and solving the needs of women and to be patient and responsive, allowing the recipients of care to evaluate and inform the process. The importance of disseminating findings through speaking and publication cannot be overrated.

Summary of key points

- It has been established beyond reasonable doubt that physiologically breast milk is the ideal food for human babies. However there are a number of factors that influence the reasons why women who wish to breastfeed are unable to do so. A key responsibility of the midwife is to develop and maintain effective skills which support the practice of breastfeeding.
- Many women who wish to breastfeed 'give up' while in hospital or while still being visited by the midwife at home. This means that when midwifery help is at its most accessible, the sharpest decline in breastfeeding is seen. Almost all the reasons given by mothers as to why they give up can be attributed to incorrectly attaching the baby at the breast. These observations suggest that at present both mothers

and midwives are insufficiently knowledgeable and skilled in this area.

- Midwifery education for both students and qualified staff on the subject of breastfeeding should be under constant review and given effective coverage in both the classroom and clinical practice, with linkage between the two to avoid inconsistent and conflicting ideas being passed on to mothers.
- Sometimes a breastfeeding policy is instituted in an attempt to avoid some of the problems of conflicting advice. However these vary tremendously around the country and many are not consistent with available research, sometimes actively hindering the establishment of successful breastfeeding.
- Any breastfeeding promotion and education must encompass examination of the attitudes of everyone involved in order to be successful.
- If a cyclical approach to learning breastfeeding is used the activity can be developed, evaluated and then further developed. Participants may also develop 'sustaining breastfeeding' workshops to continue their learning, which can then follow a continuous cyclical pattern into the future.
- Breastfeeding workshops for mothers and midwives together have been designed and implemented by the authors in order to build on the skills of the midwife and effectively cascade these to pregnant women and newly delivered mothers.
- Evaluation of the breastfeeding workshops has demonstrated that workshop attendees developed greater confidence in breastfeeding. The mothers breastfed for longer than a control group of mothers who did not attend a workshop, and the midwives as well as increasing their knowledge, noted that they needed to spend less time postnatally with women who had attended a workshop.
- The Breastfeeding Workshop package can be used in different countries and cultures, where practitioners can made adaptations to it to suit the circumstances in which it is used.
- Evaluation of such a project should come from all participants (consumers and health professionals) and findings should inform the process as it develops further.

References

Aston, J. and Bates, C. 1996: Towards a gender analysis of breastfeeding. *British Journal of Midwifery* 4(1), 5.

Clifton, A. and Long, L. 1990: The Bloomsbury Breastfeeding Workshop evaluation project. Unpublished paper.

Department of Health 1993: *Changing childbirth. Report of the Expert Maternity Group.* London: HMSO.

Dykes, F. 1995: Valuing breastfeeding in midwife education. *British Journal of Midwifery* 3(10), 544.

Garforth, S. and Garcia, J. 1989: Breastfeeding policies in practice – 'no wonder they get confused'. *Midwifery* 5, 75–83.

Green, J., Kitzinger, J. and Coupland, V. 1990: Stereotypes of childbearing women: a look at some evidence. *Midwifery* 6, 125–32.

Jamieson, L. 1990: Breastfeeding knowledge shared in a midwife mother partnership. *Proceedings of the 22nd ICM Conference*, Kobe, Japan, pp. 196–7.

Jamieson, L. 1995: Educating for successful breastfeeding. *British Journal of Midwifery* 3(10), 535.

Lawrence, R. 1994: *Breastfeeding*. St Louis: Mosby-Year Book.

Long, L. 1995: Breastfeeding Workshops: a focus on knowledge, skills and attitudes. *British Journal of Midwifery* 3(10), 450.

Maher, V. 1992: *The anthropology of breastfeeding*. Oxford: Berg Publishers.

Minchin, M. 1989: *Breastfeeding matters*. Australia: Alma Publications.

Palmer, G. 1988: *The politics of breastfeeding*. London: Pandora Press.

Raphael-Leff, J. 1990: *The Psychological processes of childbearing*. London: Chapman and Hall.

UKCC (UK Central Council for Nursing, Midwifery and Health Visiting) 1994: *The future of professional practice – the Council's standards for education and practice following registration*. Position statement on policy and implementation. London: UKCC.

UNICEF 1994: *UK baby friendly initiative. Self-appraisal: a step towards baby friendly designation*. London: UNICEF.

White, A., Freeth, S. and O'Brien, M. 1992: *Infant feeding* 1990. London: HMSO.

Wilby, L. 1995: The emotional consequences of breastfeeding failure. *British Journal of Midwifery* 3(10), 538.

15

The challenge of mental health promotion

Margaret Adams

The need for physical health promotion during the 'maternalizatum' – a behavioural term used by Prince and Adams (1987) to cover the four episodes of pregnancy, childbirth, puerperium and early motherhood – has become a major priority this century. Mortality and morbidity of both mother and baby have been dramatically reduced. The need for promotion of mental health around childbirth has, however, been less obvious. This chapter is an attempt to redress this situation.

Problems of definition

Health is compromised when the dynamic balance of an individual's makeup fails to adapt to a constantly changing external or internal environment. Nowhere is this balance so finely tuned as in the realm of mental health and nowhere is it so far reaching in the effects of its breakdown. Any upset in the mental health of a woman around childbirth will not only affect the woman, but her husband/partner, family and her whole social setting.

As discussed in Chapter 1, the dilemma of knowing how to define and interpret 'normal' health has been a subject of debate for centuries. Mental health is even more difficult to define. A wide range of emotional and behavioural responses can be seen in people reacting to similar events or circumstances. Cultural factors and the social context will further complicate these reactions and their interpretation. It may be easier therefore, in practical terms to look at a definition of mental illness, the reverse of health. Kendall and Zealley (1993) describe this as disorders in memory, perception, cognition, mood and will.

Historical overview of mental health problems following childbirth

Mental ill-health following childbirth was first described as 'illness' in the mid-nineteenth century by, among others, a doctor called Marcé. So many and varied are the 'signs and symptoms' that there was little agreement over the name of the condition. It is now frequently referred to as postnatal illness, puerperal disorder, puerperal depression (PPD) or post-natal depression (PND). Within this framework general agreement has been reached that there are four separate entities: the baby blues, post-natal depression (PND) (which may include neuroses), and puerperal psychoses. Recently, post-traumatic stress syndrome (PSD) following childbirth has been added to the discussion.

Although some level of agreement has been reached after years of debate there are still many people who dispute that these conditions can be classed as illnesses, no brain pathology having been found to account for the manifestations. In the last century, philosophers considered that mental illness was a moral issue and suggested that they would be the most suitable people to manage the sufferers. Other interested profession-als then entered the debate, such as social scientists and psychologists, whose disciplines were developed in the earlier part of this century. They have been keen to explore joint perspectives with midwives and psychia-trists. As a result, following an international conference, the Marcé Society was formed in June 1980. This brought together many interested parties and contributed to the level of agreement regarding this previously ill-defined and confusing state.

Today, social scientists have put forward an alternative model to the medical one. They suggest that social factors, rather than an individual's biological makeup, are more important. Some have suggested that PND is a realistic response to birth and its subsequent stress (Elliot, 1985). The psychologist Nicholson (1990) suggests that a model of loss (of former identity, etc.) and bereavement may be more appropriate. Katherine Paradice (1995), also a lecturer in psychology, suggested, like Ussher (1992), that it could be considered a normal response to motherhood and even 'an adaptive process ... to grieve for her lost self and to make the transition to motherhood'. In her conclusion she states that women do not want to be seen as 'victims of their hormones'. Some feminists are convinced that women are overrepresented in mental health statistics because the patriarchal system has labelled them as weak and vulnerable (Thurtle, 1995). This view does not appear to be supported by anecdotal evidence from Carol Dix (1987) and Susanna Dalton. The latter, quoted by S. Allot (1996), said on being told she had PND, 'Thank God for that; if there's a name for it there's got to be a cure'. According to Dennerstein *et al.* (1989) and Green (1990b) there is an association between antenatal and postnatal mental health. Midwives giving continuity of care are in an ideal position to recognize 'at risk' factors early and set up appropriate strategies to prevent mental health disorders (Kumar *et al.*, 1995).

The effects of mental health loss

On mother/infant interaction

There are many reasons for delayed attachment to a baby in those mothers who appear to be in a 'normal' state of mental health. Such reasons include the separation of the mother and baby immediately after birth, the 'wrong' sex or a baby with an untoward appearance, particularly when some facial abnormality is apparent. The birth of a baby with Down's syndrome, for example, does sometimes lead to its rejection either temporarily or permanently. However, problems often occur in mother/infant interaction as a result of mental health disorder.

The studies performed which explore mothers' perceptions of their newborns are small and limited to date. They also have considerable methodological limitations according to Murray (1988). Many of the data were derived from reports of women who were suffering mental ill-health, which would have coloured their perceptions of the baby. However newborn babies show rapid adaptation to a human environment and have the capacity actively to seek and regulate a response from the closest consistent caretaker, usually the mother. This exchange of responses with a second person facilitates progress developmentally, particularly with verbal communication so essential for entry to the adult world.

Can the conclusion be reached that the mental health of the mother is necessary for normal progress? Studies of pairs behaviours of mother and infant have confirmed earlier findings (Field *et al.*, 1990) that motherese (infant-directed speech) was less well-adapted to the infant's behaviour where the mother was suffering from mental ill-health (Bettes, 1988). Stein *et al.* (1991) conducted a study to see whether the effects of depression on the mother–infant relationship continue after the mother's recovery. This study looked at three groups of mothers, forty-nine in each: (1) those who had been unwell in the first year and were still depressed at 19 months, (2) mothers who had now recovered, and (3) those who were deemed 'normal'. A significant association was found between maternal depression and a reduced quality of mother–child interaction at 19 months after delivery. The association still persisted, although less positively, in those who had recovered by 19 months.

Social and marital problems are often associated with depression, and these appear to be the most important factors in poor mother–child interaction. The researchers comment that there was quite considerable variation in the depressed mothers groups. Some were nevertheless warm, and related well with their children, but this warmth was reduced in those who had ongoing severe social and marital dissatisfactions.

Beck (1995a) did a meta-analysis of nineteen studies, mainly quantitative, to find out the magnitude of the effects of PND on mother–infant interaction in the first year. Her results indicate a moderate to large adverse affect on the mother–infant interaction.

According to psychotherapist Joan Raphael-Leff (1991), a depressed mother is not available to her baby for interaction, as shown in the studies already mentioned. Long-term follow-up suggests that children of depressed mothers will have low levels of attention, concentration and other behavioural problems, often exacerbated by parental marital problems (Mills *et al.*, 1985; Caplan *et al.*, 1989).

There can, however, be more serious effects leading to deep hostility and determination to get rid of an unwanted baby by infanticide. Neonaticide, where the baby is killed within 24 hours of its delivery, is not usually associated with mental illness according to a review of the literature by Resnick (1969, 1970). However, where there is filicide (the baby is killed more than 24 hours after its birth), there is usually acute loss of mental health.

On father and family

Where a mother is unhappy, the father may feel confused and have difficulty in adapting to parenthood himself. Other siblings may increase the problems by showing aggression or regression as the family focuses on the new baby. These in turn may cause further unhappiness in the mother who is the central figure in the family's well-being. Riley (1995) comments that it is already a critical, sensitive time for family members. Both parents are trying to adapt to their lifestyle changes and relationship. If in employment the father is likely to be under pressure in his job as in many professions more work is now expected from fewer people.

His position may be insecure in the current economic climate. The woman's income may reduce or disappear and he may therefore be in an adverse financial situation, while home responsibilities may increase.

Ballard *et al.* (1994) report that 9 per cent of fathers were found to be depressed 6 weeks after a new baby's birth, and 5.4 per cent by 6 months. They were significantly more likely to have this condition if the partner was also depressed. Where a woman suffers from a puerperal psychosis and is admitted to a psychiatric unit, Harvey and McGrath (1988) found 40 per cent of their partners had 'psychiatric morbidity' compared with 4 per cent in controls. This in turn may delay the mother's recovery and affect the child or children's development (Murray *et al.*, 1991). This will increase the likelihood that some men may need counselling or treatment to enable them to support the family. The effect on the father of postnatal depression had been largely overlooked by researchers, health care professionals and the media.

Disorders in mental health

Disorders in the mental health of mothers can thus be seen to have a detrimental effect on the life of the whole family. In order to see how health can be promoted, mental health disorders need to be explored for their indicators, incidence and causes. The medical field, from which the bulk of studies have come, have used a 'scientific' or experimental approach to research. It is therefore not surprising to discover inconsistencies in the findings, as a qualitative approach would seem more appropriate. Since reported illness is of low incidence, the numbers used are small and 'normality' is difficult to define. Diagnosed psychiatric or mental illness still carries social stigma leading to a reluctance to seek help (McIntosh, 1993). Due to reluctance in admitting to emotional problems, only one-quarter of the 60 per cent of women who reported at least 2 weeks of a depressed mood in the first 9 months after delivery, consulted any health professional. Such reluctance is noted by Brockington and Cox-Roper (1988) in that 'PND fails to reach the threshold of referral'. This leads to it being a hidden, frightening disease in the homes and hearts of sufferers.

As well as the underreporting of the illness, Sherr (1995) considers that the measurements to diagnose and define these conditions are both crude and subjective, relying heavily on individual judgement. The condition is often not recognized by health care professionals according to Dix (1987). In an anonymous article in *Midwives Chronicle* a midwife describes her own experience of delayed diagnosis (Anonymous, 1993). She had great regret that it was not recognized sooner so that support could have been offered to her family.

Paradice (1995) brings an alternative view and suggests that PND should cease to be seen as an abnormal condition, but should be seen instead as a normal and understandable response to motherhood. Presumably she is not considering puerperal psychosis in this statement. Comport (1987) indicates that this is not a new view and suggests that the assumption that 'motherhood equals madness' carries the seeds of self-fulfilling prophesy and trivializes the disturbing 'real illness'.

Overview of types and incidence of mental health disorders following childbirth

The blues

Mood fluctuation is very common in new mothers. It is characterized by considerable emotional lability and is especially likely to occur as a result of insensitive professional or social contact. The mother is particularly sensitive to comments which reflect on her ability to feed her baby, and when there is conflicting advice. The 'blues' have been likened to severe pre-menstrual tension (PMT) (Riley, 1995). The condition is said to occur in 50–70 per cent of all mothers and usually lasts less than 48 hours. It is not often recognized that, when severe, it may presage the appearance of PND.

Postnatal depression (PND)

The onset of this state may be insidious and occurs usually within 2–6 weeks after delivery. A mother suffering PND will usually have insight into her state but may hide or disguise her feelings for fear of being 'labelled'. The condition will usually last 4–6 weeks if referred and treated with counselling and/or antidepressant drugs, but up to and exceeding a year if not (Kendall and Zealley, 1993). Since the effects are so detrimental to the infant and family, it is vital that the condition is recognized and treated as early as possible. The significant signs that indicate probable PND are listed in Table 15.1.

Puerperal psychosis

This condition is usually characterized by lack of insight into the disorder and by beliefs that are not founded in reality. It may start in a similar manner to 'the blues' but confusion, and severe insomnia, with a period of restlessness rapidly follow. The condition, which may last 6–12 weeks, usually requires admission to a mother and baby unit to ensure that the baby is cared for and not at risk (Kendall and Zealley, 1993). Treatment with drugs can involve neuroleptics, antidepressents and/or lithium, and

Table 15.1 Signs of postnatal depression

Sleep disturbance – easily masked by the baby needing night feeds
Acute anxiety – usually over the well-being of the baby
Inability to cope with daily living
Self-blame as she feels a less competent mother than she thinks she should be.
    She may compare herself unfavourably with her own mother and with other
    mothers she encounters (Kendall and Zealley, 1993)
Lapses of memory or concentration and irritability may contribute to a
    generally low mood
Lack of appetite and libido may occur, so adversely affecting the father
Lack of confidence in her handling of the baby, whom she may feel is not
    feeding, sleeping or behaving as it should
Fear that she may harm the baby

---

the need for support from carers is required to ensure that drugs are taken as prescribed. Counselling and rarely electroconvulsive therapy (ECT) may be resorted to when little progress is seen in carefully selected women, particularly when life-threatening depression is also present (for instance the woman is refusing to eat).

The worldwide incidence of puerperal psychosis is 0.1–0.2 per cent – that is rate of admission to mental hospital expressed as a proportion of total births (Kumar, 1990; Riley, 1995). The condition can occur in those who already have a history of psychosis. Of these, 50 per cent are likely to have a non-puerperal relapse (Marks *et al.*, 1991). In those who first have an episode postnatally there is a 1:2 to 1:7 chance of it re-occurring with further childbearing (Barnett, 1991). A list of signs that may include puerperal psychosis is given in Table 15.2.

Table 15.2 Signs of puerperal psychosis

Sudden mood changes with inappropriate laughter often turning to tears
Sudden excitement or sullen withdrawal
Sudden rejection of or ignoring the baby, or thinking that it is dead or
    abnormal
Paranoid ideas may occur as she perceives that others, often staff, or other
    new mothers, are trying to kill her and/or the baby. As already
    mentioned, she herself is the most likely person to do this
Delusions and/or hallucinations may be very real to her and she may
    hear voices

A dramatic situation (hypomania) can occur where the woman shows great confidence, optimism, excessive talk or actions. This may include spending all the money available to her or redecorating the whole house unnecessarily

---

Factors associated with loss of mental health

Since a mother's change in or loss of mental health has such a dramatic effect on the whole family, it is important that a midwife can pick up predisposing factors before the condition develops, so that early support can be offered. Research into these factors has led to apparently conflicting views. These have often reflected the stance of the researcher. Objectively measuring emotions, attitudes and behaviour remains a difficulty, even when using qualitative, observational or ethnographic approaches to the subject. Contributing causes have however emerged under the main categories of psychosocial factors, biological factors, psychiatric/emotional factors, obstetric/gynaecological factors and infant factors.

Psychosocial factors

Riley (1995) has gathered together a useful summary of the many and varied research studies of possible risk factors. Marital disharmony, poor social support and stressful life events have the most significant association. Other risk factors evidently need further research before conclusions can be firmly drawn. This is especially true of social class and marital status.

Relationship factor

A poor relationship with husband or partner is the most well-supported risk factor for loss of mental health for mothers in all studies except Wheatley's (1996) who, with a sample of forty-eight women, found that an understanding, supportive partner leads to depression. Two older (1970s) studies agreed with her but ten have found the opposite. Partners who have their own emotional problems were not able to give much support and the women were more likely to be depressed.

A recent American survey (Schaper *et al.*, 1994) found that marital instability was one of three factors correlating most significantly with elevated Edinburgh Postnatal Depression Scores (EPDS) which can be found in Cox and Holden (1994).

Social support

A large longitudinal study by Williams *et al.* (1981) in the general field of mental health, came to these conclusions:

- Effective social support systems predict improvements in mental health over a period of time.
- Negative life events and physical limitations predict a deterioration in mental health over time.

These results suggest the need for a support system for childbearing women.

Stern and Kruckona (1983), amongst others, have suggested that PND is a syndrome of modern Western society. An industrialized society, it is argued, brings limited community support with its nuclear and often single-parent families. A study by Thorpe *et al.* (1992) looked at the effects of life events and social support within a modern society in the UK and a more traditional society in Greece which, although just starting its transition to modern society, still has close knit family groupings. In the UK sample, emotional well-being of mothers had, as its predictors, social support and the partner's emotional well-being. Although the Greek women perceived less support, this did not affect their emotional well-being, but stressful life circumstances were reported to have a detrimental effect. Three of these circumstances related to the extended family. It may be that living with parents or in-laws is a source of stress rather than support. These findings are tentative as shared meanings vary between cultures, and there was no Greek comparative control group.

Cox (1988) carried out a controlled trial in another traditional society, Uganda, which gives special childbirth rituals (rites of passage) to new mothers. He found the incidence of PND was 10 per cent in both Uganda and Scotland, but he does however acknowledge some weaknesses in the study. Evidently more research is needed in this area. However, the incidence of postpartum psychosis is unaffected by culture and has been shown through data and historical evidence to have remained unchanged over 150 years (Kumar, 1990).

Nicholson (1990) found, in a small qualitative study, that 'the degree and quality of support in the early months of mothering was probably the single most crucial factor accounting for emotional stability'. He suggests that the concept of PND should be re-examined as it is more akin to the normal grief and loss process and possibly part of the postnatal scene. However, this does not explain why it should happen after subsequent pregnancies when the lifestyle has already changed and loss of independence has already taken place.

Other sociological surveys have also shown that for emotional well-being the mother needs a confidante. New mothers may have lost colleagues and friends from work if recently employed and will need to find new friends, a further source of possible stress.

Relationship with own mother

Raphael-Leff (1991) considers that this relationship is of central importance in the maternalizatum. She reports a sadness and feelings of deprivation where a woman had lost her own mother during childhood from death, divorce or separation. Some of her observations of new mothers showed they did not have as much interaction with their babies as women who still had a mother. The lack of a role model can also affect their behaviour towards the babies. Murray *et al.* (1995) found that postnatal depression was more likely to occur in women who had a poor relationship with their mother, whereas in other forms of depression within a control group there was no such definite association.

Biological factors

Hormones – oestrogen/progesterone

There have been few studies carried out on these factors. Until 1996 only one study (Henderson *et al.*, 1991) found a correlation between oestrogen and PND whereas three earlier studies did not. A controlled trial of sixty-four women with severe non-psychotic PND was carried out by Gregoire *et al.* (1996) and the results indicated that there was a rapid (within first month) rise in mood in those who had transdermal oestrogen, unlike those who had placebo patches. The women volunteers were only those not breastfeeding or on oral contraceptives, and were within 18 months of delivery. Half the treated group had had conventional antidepressant drugs for at least 6 weeks, without any benefits seen. The results are convincing but further research is needed as soon as possible, (as indicated by Gregoire) into minimum effective dosage, length of treatment and whether oestrogen has wider antidepressant properties. There is also the question of whether it can be used in those who are breastfeeding. It is too early to use oestrogen as a first-line treatment, as Gregoire appears to have conducted the only controlled trial into its use to date.

The use of progesterone has been vigorously commended and used by Dalton (1985) with little sound scientific evidence to support its use. Van der Meer *et al.* (1984) found that this hormone had no more effect than a placebo.

Thyroid hormones

Mood changes occur with both hypo- and hyperthyroidism. According to Riley (1995) 20 per cent of postnatal women have mild dysfunction of the thyroid. Most commonly a degree of hyperthyroidism occurs between 1 and 4 months after delivery, and hypothyroidism after the fourth month. A small number of such women will suffer from PND (Harris, 1993).

Psychiatric/emotional factors

Watson *et al.* (1984) showed that of those few (6–14 per cent) women who have had previous psychiatric history, 60 per cent showed signs of PND at 6 weeks postpartum. The risk of a recurrence of PND varied from 25 to 75 per cent. The evidence from other studies is somewhat less clear.

There is stronger evidence that 'the blues' are related to PND. When this condition is severe, about half the women will continue into PND, according to Dennerstein *et al.* (1989), and Hannah *et al.* (1992).

A qualitative study by Green (1990b) has looked at factors correlating with emotional well-being. This large-scale prospective study looked at women's feelings of well-being rather than depression. The response rate was good, increasing the survey's validity. Green found a strong association between ante- and postnatal mood. Those women who were happy to be pregnant remained happy in the puerperium. Unhappiness was increased by feelings of lack of control in labour, lack of involvement in decision-making and feelings that interventions were not right for them. The 'unhappy' women felt fear and helplessness and saw staff as 'rushed' and 'bossy'. Dennerstein *et al.* (1989) also found antenatal mood a major determinant of postnatal mood.

Obstetric/gynaecological factors

Some research has been carried out to investigate the connection between various obstetric and gynaecological factors and mental ill-health. Caesarean section performed under general anaesthesia appears to carry the greatest risk of subsequent PND according to Fisher *et al.* (1990). Parity appears to be only a risk in a young woman having her third or subsequent baby. Generally, obstetric interventions such as induction, forceps delivery, etc. do not appear to carry a risk unless, as already mentioned, the woman did not feel them to be right for her (Green, 1990b).

In 1996, however, Dr Fiona Blake (1996) reported at a conference that post-traumatic stress disorder following childbirth is considerably under-diagnosed. Helen Allot (1996), an obstetrician, runs a postdelivery stress clinic where she sees women who have had a psychologically traumatic delivery and cannot face a future pregnancy. Dr Janet Menage (1996) studied 500 women, of whom one-fifth had had a distressing obstetric or gynaecological procedure. She considered 1.5 per cent could be diagnosed as suffering from post-traumatic stress disorder (PSD).

A woman who has had an unexplained stillbirth, neonatal or cot death is likely to suffer anxiety in her next pregnancy with the possibility of PND following it (Clarke and Williams, 1979). Little evidence of direct association between menstrual disorders, pre-menstrual tension, termination of pregnancy, or miscarriage, has been made (Clarke and Williams, 1979; Friedman and Gath, 1989; Field *et al.*, 1990).

Some other factors, such as fear or difficulty in pregnancy and breast-feeding, have also been studied without any clear conclusions.

Infant factors

Even when newborn, babies vary in both appearance and behaviour. Some babies, for instance, are 'cuddly' whilst others are not (Prince and Adams, 1987). Others are placid, restless or crying, not easy to settle and so may be perceived as 'difficult'. A few of these variations can be explained by the fact that they have been ill, have an abnormality, or have received intensive care. Recently however, attention has been focused on the effect that variations in behaviour may have on maternal mood (Crockenburg, 1986). This study, amongst others, assessed babies who were more than 2 months old and could have been affected themselves by having a depressed mother. Murray *et al.* (1996) carried out a complex study with mothers who were either at high or low risk of depression. Their babies were assessed at one week of life, when relatively little exposure to their mother's mood had occurred. In the 'high-risk' group of mothers who became depressed, 34 per cent of cases were considered to be associated with infant factors. Those factors included neonatal irritability and poor motor function, which could not be explained by obstetric complications such as 'fetal distress'. Unexpectedly, poor motor function had the more marked effect on low- as well as high-risk groups. Even a slight degree of this malfunction interferes with the eye-to-eye contact so essential in mother/baby interaction.

Mental health promotion

It is clear from all the studies so far examined that no single cause for PND has yet been discovered. There are, however, various factors that are associated with the condition or conditions which can be encompassed under the generic term of postnatal illness.

Prevention of mental ill-health is vital, as it has been estimated by Ball (1989) that a conservative estimate of 60 000 families are disturbed or affected by it at any one time. Prevention is better than cure, as with the latter, however early it is instituted, disruption of the family will have already started. Cox (1989) asks the question 'Can PND be prevented?'. He concludes that since no single cause has been discovered, there can be no single cure, but early recognition of 'risk' factors may lead to prevention of ill-health. These factors and others are summarized in Figs 15.1 and 15.2.

Detection of risk factors by the midwife and midwifery strategies

The midwife is in an ideal position, according to Kumar *et al.* (1995), to detect risk factors during pregnancy. The first or subsequent encounter with an 'at risk' pregnant woman may or may not reveal many of these rather personal factors. Much will depend on the way in which the first interview is conducted.

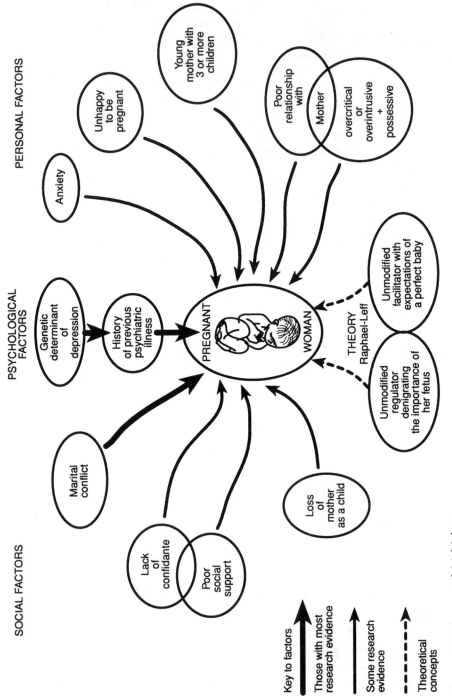

Figure 15.1 Antenatal 'risk' factors

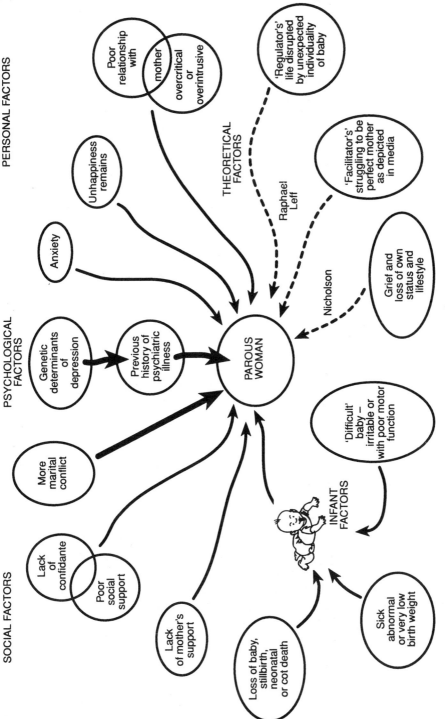

Figure 15.2 Antenatal plus postnatal 'risk' factors

The midwife's attitudes

All human beings develop attitudes (Lambert and Lambert, 1964), starting with an initial adjustment as children, to their social environment.
This starts in the family, with parental pressure, then at school or college
more influence becomes exerted over attitude development. The media
pours views, opinions and 'facts' into us so that some attitudes become
'fixed' and develop into prejudice. Some of these influence how we react
when first meeting a woman whose culture, ethnicity, class, habits or
social functioning we have already pre-judged. We need to be aware of
our own prejudice so that we can have an open, non-judgemental, unbiased approach, in order that each woman feels able to disclose to us
very personal information where this is appropriate.

A series of experiential workshops, facilitated by the author between
1988 and 1992 as part of a continuing education programme, revealed
much about some midwives' attitudes. It was discovered that there were
certain women we did not like caring for. A modified nominal group
technique was used so that individual midwives' views were only known
to a small group. The commonest disliked women were those perceived
as dirty or smelly, professionals like teachers and lawyers, those who
were rude and aggressive, those without a sense of humour or seen as
inflexible and those who failed to recognize the status of the midwife.

The most liked were women who were clean, cheerful, open-minded,
cooperative, ordinary, good communicators and those who were appre-
ciative! Those who were disadvantaged or with mental health disability
problems did not appear to raise strong feelings either way. The groups
were experienced midwives from widely differing cultures and ethnic
groups. Most participants acknowledged that they had become aware of
their own attitudes and hopefully would become more socially sensitive.
These findings showed some commonalities with an Australian nursing
study by Roberts (1984).

The midwives' interpersonal skills

According to Methven (1989), many midwives have had little education
in interviewing clients, where the purpose is to obtain a holistic view of a
woman. She discovered that the emphasis is still focused mainly on
physical and medical facts and little in the psychosocial area. Both are
important so that both physical and mental complications may be
avoided.

The quality of the interview may be enhanced by the use of the
Midwifery Process approach. This was pioneered by Adams *et al.* (1981)
and Bryar (1987), and further studied by Methven. Communication and
basic 'counselling' skills, however, are the most vital ingredients in
building up a rapport with the woman, so she will be free to talk about
her feelings and emotions and to reveal details, which she may fear

would 'label' her, such as a previous psychiatric history, provided she is assured of confidentiality.

Human communication is a very complex process and, according to Pease (1974), a large component is non-verbal. This non-verbal communication (NVC) is 'given off' as described by Goffman (1982) and Pease (1974). It will be received and interpreted by the participants before a word can be said. This is especially true of attitudes which are interpreted in the light of each participant's own background. For instance, busyness or tiredness can be seen as disinterest or lack of concern, which immediately affects the two-way communication process. An interaction between woman and midwife should occur as a conversation between equals, as advocated by the *Changing childbirth* report (Department of Health, 1993b).

Questioning is an important skill and it is essential to distinguish between 'open' and 'closed' questions. Only non-directive open questions encourage a person to express their feelings. Methven (1989) studied forty antenatal interviews and found just three questions which were open. The vast majority were closed, which, according to Macleod Clark (1981), powerfully control or block the development of a conversation. Even when open questions were asked in Methven's study, a direct question would follow before the woman could reply.

One of the open questions used in the midwifery Process approach prior to the booking interview was how a woman felt when she realized she was pregnant: eighteen women said they were very pleased, nine had mixed feelings and thirteen were shocked, 'scared', 'horrified' or 'shattered'. By the booking interview they had somewhat changed in their views with: fifteen still being pleased, seventeen with mixed feelings and eight still not happy. This useful question was not seen as intrusive, direct or embarrassing as would 'Was your pregnancy planned or not?'.

Screening for at risk depression factors brings another challenge. Clearly it is not ethical to discover a factor and take no action, and a midwife should be able to refer a woman directly to the liaison psychiatrist or community psychiatric nurse (CPN) or to a qualified counsellor or psychotherapist if wanted. Such a maternity psychiatric service continues to run at Kings College Hospital and has been described by Appleby *et al.* (1989). Since 1989 the Brierley Midwifery Practice has been set up to give care to those with and without mental health problems. Women with such problems are not therefore 'labelled' as having psychiatric care, as it is seen as normal antenatal care (Kumar *et al.*, 1995; Meyer and Wallace, 1995). Ninety-eight per cent of this group of women have had continuity of care from one of three midwives right through pregnancy, delivery and up to 28 days postnatally. The midwives provide stability and security to those who lack both in their lives. They have monthly meetings with a senior psychiatric registrar and the perinatal consultant as well as the obstetrician, who is available for advice. They themselves have had no additional 'counselling training' but their flexible service with support, continuity and choice of birthplace gives control to the women. Assessment of whether there is a reduced rate of PND has not yet taken place but anecdotal evidence suggests that both midwives and mothers find the practice very satisfactory. Riley (1995) commends this type of approach, as it is her opinion that women would prefer to be cared for by professionals they already know, rather than being referred to a psychiatrist with all its social stigma.

Preparation for parenthood?

Some mothers and midwives may agree with the view of Paradice (1995) that PND is a normal response to motherhood. More will argue with her that women are not initially aware of the impact a new baby will have on their lives, which will never be quite the same again. She suggests that midwives, as the central carers during the maternalizatum, could do more to educate women on the nature of PND arising from the shock of the changes that a new baby will bring. McIntosh (1993) reports that this 'shock' is related to PND too, and calls for better preparation for 'the realities of motherhood'. Three-quarters of his small sample of women felt that their own view of motherhood was unrealistic and that a less glamorous view of the state needs to be presented. This would go some way to reduce the over-romantic view so often portrayed by the media and some professionals. It would help a mother who feels she is inadequate because she is not perfect, to realize that she is not abnormal in this respect. Many of the women in McIntosh's study had heard about depression during their antenatal care or classes. McIntosh acknowledges that his conclusions are tentative due to the limited sample used. However, as long ago as 1976/77 the Report on Violence to Children (Department of Health, 1978) highlighted the fact that parents do not know enough about parenting and that parentcraft education should be given more importance, as was also emphasized by Cox (1986).

This issue is still being raised. Enkin *et al.* (1995), for example, call for portrayal of more realism of the responsibility during the maternalizatum and early parenthood. Cox (1986) considers that explaining that some mothers may become depressed after childbirth is essential. He considers fear of upsetting the mother reflects the attitude of the teacher rather than the needs of women and their families. Problems of providing a realistic view of the subject to suit all mothers was also discussed in 1977 by Adams. The opinion of Niven (1992) is that effective antenatal preparation needs to be based on reality rather than reassurance. Bohn (1990), in a review of research on the subject of family conflict, estimates that 1 in 50 of all pregnant women will be beaten, making the incidence higher than that of placenta previa or gestational diabetes. The worst attacks, according to Dobash and Dobash (1987), include conflict, firstly arising from sexual jealousy, and secondly over expectations concerning help with domestic work.

It is not surprising that a new mother feels overwhelmed by all the baby-related chores such as dirty washing, etc. on top of all the usual domestic chores. It is often suggested there have been considerable changes in the role of men accompanying the changed social role of women, but perhaps this more recent research shows less change than the media depicts. Fathers may expect to participate in the care of the children, but perhaps only in the more rewarding aspects.

Discussions could be encouraged at parentcraft, when men are present, on the effects the new baby can have on the couple and family. Stress management could also be included so that stress can be alleviated without untoward anger. Dix (1987) suggests making an antenatal plan for those who have had PND once and intend to avoid it if at all possible. This could form a very useful tool for discussion between all potential parents, as they are helped to think through the radical life changes and effects on the family that the baby will bring.

Wilson (1990), an experienced antenatal educator, considers this is often an neglected area, in spite of the Court report (Department of Health, 1976) which called for clearer guidance and advice for parents and for the father to enter into full parental partnership. Often classes have more emphasis on the knowledge that midwives and others think the parents need. More involvement with participation is still needed, with movement away from formal lectures. Adults appreciate experiential learning, but facilitating this learning can bring an uncomfortable feeling to inexperienced teachers, according to Wilson (1990). In a small survey, she found that out of twenty-eight midwives teaching parentcraft

- 82 per cent started teaching before attending a teaching course,
- 46 per cent started without any tuition in the theories of learning or in practical class planning,
- 29 per cent had had no tuition during their training or since, and
- 32 per cent only attended a course *after* they commenced the teaching post.

Black (1986) found a similar picture in her study. Now that there is a trend for all midwives in a team to teach parentcraft, one wonders whether the situation could become worse, unless they have all had a teaching module in the Diploma or Degree midwifery course or that many midwives now attend or have attended an ENB approved teaching course and have put the theory into practice since completing it. Prince and Adams, as long ago as 1977, commented that midwives lacked opportunities to develop their teaching skills and that students then often lacked the depth of knowledge demanded by our sophisticated society's demands. They commented that furthermore, health visitors who do receive training to educate, often lack the wealth of practical experience needed for a realistic preparation for childbirth.

One health visitor, Debbie Okpala (1991), who is also a midwife, set up a small project with a physiotherapist and a community midwife. The purpose was to investigate why ten women with 'at risk' factors for PND rejected the traditional parentcraft teaching where information was imparted by lectures and videos. In an attempt to discover the reasons for this rejection she used two antenatal questionnaires, the first of which was to discover the factors that could interfere with a healthy pregnancy, either on a physical, emotional or social level. The second was on 'feelings' and was designed to detect potential areas of family conflict in order to enhance positive attitudes and find ways to cope. The purpose was to reveal the individual needs of the participating women so that they could be discussed amongst their peers. Myths were corrected, symptoms explained, and support enlisted at classes which could help after the delivery. She was able to refer any 'threatening conditions' identified to appropriate agencies. Discussions on how to handle partners' feelings and to involve other children to minimize sibling rivalry or rejection resulting from the impending birth were included. The group became the Enterprise Mother and Baby Group and continued for 18 months instead of the usual cessation of parentcraft sessions after the birth. One of the reasons for the success of this small group was probably that it was democratically led and woman-centred, whilst using and valuing all the group members' contributions. No doubt considerable listening skills were used to perceive the woman's non-verbal as well as verbal and written communication. The group also continued after the births so that there was continuity of support.

Reducing anxiety in the antenatal period

Watson *et al.* (1984) found that undue anxiety is associated with PND. Some causes of this anxiety can be seen in Fig. 15.1, and include reactivation of post-traumatic events associated with previous loss of a fetus or baby (Tylden, 1990). A number of older studies have reported increased anxiety during pregnancy (Elliot *et al.*, 1983; Condon, 1987). Sharp (1989) found that twenty-two out of thirty-two women with PND at 3 months after birth, had been depressed during pregnancy.

New technology has introduced another set of anxiety-provoking issues, including that of prenatal screening and diagnosis. There is some evidence to suggest that those who accept such tests are already more anxious than those who do not, and that it is not the tests *per se* causing the anxiety (Marteau *et al.*, 1992b; Green *et al.*, 1994). Many women do not realize that the purpose of the screening tests is to detect an abnormality (Abramsky, 1994). Marteau *et al.* (1992a) observed the way in which women were encouraged to have the screening tests by the way the tests were presented by the staff. They found that the test results were only relayed to the parents if they were positive ie the result was abnormal and there was little explanation given that, even if a test came back negative, a perfect baby was not guaranteed. The issue of subsequent termination of pregnancy when a test was positive was not discussed by all the obstetricians and midwives with the women before the screening test. The questions of what constitutes adequate pre-test counselling is discussed fully by Abramsky (1994). A major element is to help the couple to make a decision which is suitable for them, having considered the consequences and acceptability to them. Abramsky (1994) considers that this 'very definitely does not involve counsellors giving advice which is essentially what *they* think *they* would do in the situation. What the counsellors would do is entirely irrelevant. It is not their baby and they will not have to live with the consequences of any decisions which are made.' She acknowledges that this non-directive approach is sharply in contrast with other medical areas where patients are advised what they should do. She notes that it is difficult for health professionals, like doctors or midwives, who are used to advice-giving (directive counselling), to be non-directive in these circumstances.

Abramsky (1994) also studied counselling practices prior to amniocentesis in one region in the UK. It was found that the time a senior doctor or midwife spent 'counselling' on a routine antenatal visit, was between 5 and 15 minutes. The fact that the cell culture could fail was mentioned in less than half the units studied, as was the possibility, should abnormality be found, of having a midtrimester termination. The fact that there was a possibility of a false negative resulting from amniocentesis was not mentioned, nor that chromosome abnormalities other than Down's syndrome could also be discovered.

It is evident that some 'counsellors' did not listen to the counsellee's views, beliefs or values. 'Listening is a skill that some people seem to have in abundance and other people seem to lack in equal abundance!' Abramsky comments that it can, however, be learned, but many health workers finish their training without the ability really to listen. These comments again emphasize the need for midwives to learn and practise communication skills. These are helpful in reducing the severe anxiety that some women have as a response to prenatal screening, as reported by Green (1990a) and so avoid extra stress on those 'at risk' of PND.

Reducing anxiety during labour

The management of labour has changed dramatically over the last 20 years, from medical and technical domination, to considerable attention being paid to psychological aspects of care. Humanizing the environment has been used to create one which is more like home. However, one study in The Netherlands by Kleiverda *et al.* (1991) found that neither giving birth at home nor voluntarily giving birth in hospital was related to a woman's postpartum well-being. Well-being during her pregnancy was, however, related to her postnatal well-being and not the subjective experiences surrounding delivery. Altering furnishings in an institution ignores the fact that it is people who create humanistic care of 'being with' as well as doing, for women, according to McKay (1991).

In Green's (1990b) study, women who were unhappy to be pregnant became more so during childbirth, so particular attention needs to be paid to identifying these women so that they may feel more positive about the event and not perceive midwives as 'rushed' or 'bossy' but 'informative'. Adams (1989), using an ethnographic approach, explored a small number of scenarios of midwives' communication with primigravidae during the second stage of labour using video recordings. It emerged that the women who felt most satisfied with information given, and had their questions answered, were those who had an Educating/Encouraging (E/E) midwife. Those who were least satisfied – less than half – had a Directing (D) midwife, who also retained control. The E/E midwife passed on her knowledge so that the woman appeared more in control of her labour. Other properties of these conceptual models were that the D group gave minimum information, and did not reply to, or discouraged questions. The E/E midwife was seen as friendly and informative. Questions were encouraged and answered honestly. The need for further development of interpersonal skills was highlighted and also the need for a language which would enable midwife and client to share meanings about the process of labour.

Continuity of care and carer has been seen as a great assistance in the social aspects of childbirth, as suggested by Prince and Adams (1987). This continuity, however, can be dispiriting to the carer if a rapport is difficult to achieve, or there is some serious complication. This can be very emotionally draining to an inexperienced midwife or one who is especially vulnerable. She may herself have had a similar complication leading to fetal or neonatal loss. All human beings find it difficult to stay alert and attentive in demanding or repetitive tasks, and should have the option of being able to have a break after 2 hours at most. The midwife will then return with a fresh approach to the situation. Helen Allot (1996) suggests that a psychologically traumatic delivery for a woman can have a profound effect on any future pregnancies and even sexual relationships. Adams (1989) agreed with Henderson (1984) 'that it is the midwife who decides the quality of care mothers experience, regardless of delivery outcome. It is up to the midwifery profession to improve this care in the matter of communication'. Action to improve communication between mother and midwife in the labour room may lead to a reduction of psychological trauma, but this is yet to be researched.

The midwife and postnatal mental health promotion

Psychiatrists, in particular Professor Kumar, who was instrumental in founding the Marcé Society, as well as Cox (1986), consider that the midwife's role is crucial to the promotion and good management of mental health. There are many opportunities to recognize women at risk and to intervene or refer those showing signs of sliding into depression after 'the blues' or with other 'at risk' factors (Fig. 15.2).

The education a midwife has received, however, may not sufficiently sensitize her to the urgent need for intervention and treatment of any disorders. There is still considerable dispute about the causes of PND, but there is almost universal agreement over the urgent need for immediate recognition leading to diagnosis and early treatment. The midwife is considered by many to be in the key position to recognize the subtle alterations in the mother's behaviour, especially in those she has cared for from early pregnancy. As well as the signs already described, Niven (1992) highlights the need to be alert to a mother who views her baby as a 'poor thing, entering an unhappy world', whilst the baby looks and behaves quite normally. It may be that the woman has projected her feelings on to the baby.

Eden (1989) studied the knowledge and management of PND by Australian midwives. It was found that PND was confused with puerperal psychosis, and the midwife's ability to manage it was, in Eden's opinion, not good. The midwives considered that their knowledge and management were associated with their lack of both time and lack of continuity in care. The latter is particularly lacking in Australia, as midwives are excluded from most antenatal care and assessment, leaving them without a baseline of individual norms from which to measure psychological and behavioural changes.

If in the UK a trend which encourages practice nurses to do antenatal care grows and develops, a similar situation could possibly arise. The resulting fragmented care would detract from mental health promotion during the maternalizatum. Selective community postnatal visits by midwives may decrease the identification of mothers who are most at risk of slipping into depression.

How competent are midwives in the UK at recognizing emotional distress? In a large survey carried out in 1987 by Ball (1989) it appeared that there was some difficulty as the midwives attributed the distress to physical comforts and breastfeeding problems. They reported 1 per cent of women as having the 'blues' but noted that 15 per cent had sleeping problems and 20 per cent were tearful! Neither doctors nor midwives, contrary to Cox's (1986) advice, took these signs into account when assessing the women. Riley (1995) suggests that the use of a checklist could be helpful. She suggests including the following questions:

- Does the mother feel she is getting enough sleep?

- Does she have a choice over nursery or rooming-in at night?
- Has she sufficient support and help at home?

Riley also warns that it is all too easy for the 'blues' to be misinterpreted as early signs of psychosis, or for psychotic signs to be ignored and not taken seriously.

What can a midwife do when she is concerned over the state of a new mother's emotions? She may not have such a well-developed maternity psychiatric liaison service as that which has been developed at Kings College Hospital. Kumar *et al.* (1995) comment that midwives may not be psychiatrists or social workers, 'but they should know someone who is'. While awaiting help from the liaison psychiatrist, community psychiatric nurse (CPN) or social worker, her listening skills can be used to good effect, as acknowledged by Holden *et al.* (1989). If time is very short, asking the woman to complete an Edinburgh Postnatal Depression Scale questionnaire can be useful and has been shown to be acceptable to mothers. An example of a question from the EPDS is 'I have felt worried and anxious for no very good reason: No, not at all/Hardly ever/Yes, sometimes/Yes, very often.' (Cox and Holden, 1994: 140). Scoring the women's answers from a provided scoring sheet will help the midwife reach a more objective decision of the woman's mental state.

The process of restoring mental health can quickly be instituted by counselling and/or antidepressant drugs. In the experience of Kumar (1990) and others, the prognosis for short- and medium-term depression is excellent, most women making a full recovery. If not treated, it may last longer than one year and be the start of a lifetime of vulnerability. There is still a high risk of recurrence after another birth.

The drugs used do carry a risk to a baby who is being breastfed. Kumar (1990) comments that all psychotropic drugs are secreted in breast milk. Riley (1995) raises a query over the quantities which will affect the baby and when the effects will occur. The risks are higher in a baby whose liver function is poor, such as in one who is jaundiced or preterm. She considers that the benefits to a mother who has only a minor degree of ill-health may outweigh the risks in some individuals. Medication is, however, absolutely essential in severe disorders, particularly chronic psychosis, where there is a risk of harm coming to the mother and/or baby. Encouragement to continue the medication is needed, as well as an understanding of its side-effects.

The postnatal period is not easy for a mother who is liable to develop PND when there is a discontinuity of health professionals (Cox, 1988). When a midwife hands over the responsibility of care to the health visitor without good liaison and without an appreciation of each others' expertize, the woman could 'drop through the net', particularly if there is interprofessional rivalry. A mother needs to know to whom she can turn when motherhood is becoming a strain and she sees motherhood or her baby in a negative light.

Dix (1987) feels that the average GP misses many cases of PND, giving out drugs without fully acknowledging that what they are seeing is indeed PND. Seeley *et al.* (1996), in an article with a psychiatrist and psychologist, comments that often in the course of routine care, PND can go undetected and the NHS has no resources to meet affected women's needs. Studies are also reviewed by Seeley, which show that health visitor interventions can detect, manage and help with mother–baby relationships.

McClary and Stokoe (1995) describe the launch of a postnatal depression strategy for PND in Oxford city. This multidisciplinary approach started with a senior nurse for health visiting, a senior midwife, a purchaser, a GP, a community psychiatric nurse and a member of the health promotion unit. A consultant psychologist and registrar in obstetric liaison psychiatry joined the group later to develop a district protocol. The purpose was to raise GPs' awareness of the input of a health visitor as the key worker, so that it could enhance the GP's own management. The strategy was to put the client in its centre and identify helpful interventions, whilst diminishing professional overlap and duplication. The health visitors were further trained in active listening skills and non-directive counselling. Since there is enthusiasm with teamwork for the project, it is hoped that the evaluation will show a good outcome for this collaborative approach.

Pitts (1995) describes a health visitor-led group approach which appears both effective and cost-efficient. She suggest that because of the serious consequences of PND, that health visitors 'should regard depressed mothers as a priority'. The mothers were assessed with the use of the EPDS scale which has been validated to detect PND (Cox *et al.*, 1987). Kumar (personal communication, 1996) stresses that although this scale is a useful tool, it should not be used to replace personal interaction.

The views of mothers experiencing PND were sought by Beck (1995b) in the USA. Several themes that illustrated their nursing care emerged from her phenomenological study. There were: (1) having sufficient knowledge of PND, (2) using astute observation and intuition to make fast accurate diagnosis, (3) providing hope that there is an end to their living nightmare, (4) giving continuity of care, (5) being empathetic and (6) referring when appropriate. Beck followed this with a study in 1996 of the mothers' own thoughts, perceptions and feelings whilst suffering PND. The results included the following:

- They felt overwhelmed by the responsibility for the baby, and terrified to be left alone with him/her.
- Some were aware they erected barriers between themselves and their baby.

- Some did not yearn for interaction with the baby and they didn't respond to its cues.
- They felt guilty about being the worst mother in the world.
- Some felt uncontrollable anger which often led to seeking help.
- Some of them strived to minimize their negative effect on the baby by making an effort to interact and also enlisted help from friends and relatives.

This study highlights the effectiveness of using phenomenological research to gain these helpful insights into the perceptions in the depressed mothers' world. It should help all carers to convey a better understanding of women when listening, so that the mothers do not feel so hopeless and isolated, but are aware of being accepted non-judgementally. This can provide a first step towards recovery.

An interesting initiative comes from Australia. Milgrom (1994) proposes an intervention programme to modify the negative influences from maternal depression on the interaction of the mother with her baby. A programme for a group of depressed mothers and their partners is described. It is called 'The Baby Happiness Understanding, Giving and Sharing (HUGS) nursing programme' and consists of six phases. In the first, a warm trusting environment is created to help parents share their feelings about pregnancy and labour, and to explore their current needs. Particular attention is paid to seeing how social support networks can be widened and how the parents can have planned time for themselves. Further phases include the promotion of physical contact with their baby, and observing and interpreting its cues. Parents are encouraged to notice how their child shows subtle expressions of personality. If these are not understood, the parents may find their responses, however well intentioned, do not meet the baby's needs, resulting sometimes in feelings of frustration and rejection. Understanding different interpretation of the baby's behaviour can often lessen these feelings. Parents are then encouraged to introduce their baby to the group by describing his or her personality. This highlights the many temperamental variants of each baby. The final phase depends on whether the group would benefit from sessions aimed at strengthening marital relationships, or whether it is needed on an individual basis. This HUGS programme can, according to Milgrom, be run by any health care professional who has experience in group facilitation, providing they have a wide knowledge of babies' psychological and motor development.

Policy recommendations

Existing midwifery services

Poor attitudes and lack of communication skills still rank highly in clients' complaints, so a midwife who has had little training in interpersonal skills can herself request experiential workshops to cover these topics. These workshops could usefully focus on listening and basic 'counselling' skills, the need for which has been identified by Davis and Fallowfield (1992) and Hutton (1994) amongst many others. The former also comment that midwives can make or mar sensitive occasions during the maternalizatum, an example being the way antenatal screening is handled. Listening is a valuable therapy for women in our care and can help us provide a confiding relationship so often missing. Jacobson *et al.* (1991) suggest that improvements in interpersonal skills should lead to 'an increase in parental satisfaction and a decrease in anxiety related to the antenatal period'.

As an alternative to the workshops, day conferences arranged by such organizations as the Marcé Society and the Institute of Psychiatry in London, are also available. The Marcé Society also provides a distance learning package *The emotional effects of childbirth* (1996).

Books may also be a useful resource for both midwife and client. Dix (1987), despite its age, and Barnett (1991) both contain useful strategies for women at risk of becoming depressed.

It has already been noted that it is important to identify possible 'at risk' women as early as possible. This will need to be done with great care and tact to avoid the woman feeling 'labelled'. If one midwife gives continuity of care, she can give priority to early exploration of women's feelings. The current trend for reducing the number of antenatal visits will not help, however, in the development of a confiding relationship.

Ongoing education should also encourage midwives to feel more confident in airing the subject of mental health in parentcraft classes, although some would argue that this is an area for the midwife 'specialist' as suggested by Page (1993). If midwives themselves have easy access to psychiatric expertise, such as in the Brierley Practice described by Meyer and Wallace (1995), it would encourage them to identify 'at risk' women more readily. In addition, it would also be helpful if they knew to whom they could refer such clients. Riley (1995) suggests that a specialist in each health district could encourage and support midwives, and involve them in a network for prevention, screening and early treatment.

Laryea (1989) suggests that in the postnatal period there is an imbalance between physical and emotional care. Furthermore, Hutton (1994) comments that new mothers are still confused by conflicting advice, especially over infant feeding which leads to considerable anxiety, one factor identified as contributing to PND. Some attempts have been made to reduce this conflict by the use of experiential workshops in which midwives are encouraged to share their expertise and practical suggestions, and discuss areas of conflicting advice to differentiate fact and unsubstantiated opinion (see Chapter 14).

Further research

Jacobson *et al.* (1991) in *The nation's health* stressed the need for further research to be carried out as well-designed studies are rather few in number. Areas suggested for investigation include the effects of temporary social support by counsellors. As far back as 1988, O'Hara and Zekoski (1988) maintained that the community needs to have a voice in the allocation of scarce governmental resources. Many midwives are making an effort to improve the care of their clients within their tight budget. Hutton (1994) suggests that the provision of new maternity units is insufficient unless staffing levels are raised. Those who control resource allocation should realize that the health of the nation's families can be seriously affected by the undetected and therefore untreated effects of PND, thus leading to expensive professional help. Prevention would be beneficial to all concerned, on a personal as well as financial level.

Services to support women

Cox in 1989 called for two community psychiatric nurses to be identified in each health district, to give essential back-up and training to midwives and health visitors. Dube (1992), one such community psychiatric nurse, makes the point that she could be involved in antenatal education, and take direct referrals from midwives as well as organizing postnatal support groups. This would short-circuit the delays in referral that are often encountered as a midwife is not often able to refer directly to a psychiatrist.

These suggestions could help to meet one target of *The health of the nation* (Department of Health, 1993a) to improve significantly the health and social functioning of mentally ill people.

Summary of key points

- The definition of mental health and its disorders is complicated and controversial. The literature commonly divides postnatal mental ill-health into postnatal depression and postnatal psychosis. More recently post-traumatic stress disorder has been suggested as an occurrence which can follow childbirth.
- Many women who have disordered mental health postnatally were also affected in pregnancy. Women who demonstrate great anxiety in pregnancy are at greater risk of postnatal depression.
- 'The blues' are common in the first few days after birth and are often described as a normal part of the transition into motherhood. However, when severe 'the blues' can act as an indication that postnatal depression may follow.

- The effects of maternal mental illness on the baby and the whole family can be profound and long term. There is considerable evidence that they continue even after the mother has recovered.
- No single factor explains loss of mental health. The factors that are most often suggested from a review of current literature on the subject are previous psychiatric problems, marital disharmony, poor social support, stressful life events, poor relationship with one's own mother, hormone imbalances, obstetric factors and infant factors.
- Effective mental health promotion may do much to prevent and alleviate suffering in society; it has been estimated that 60 000 or more families are disturbed or affected by postnatal depression at any one time.
- The midwife is in an ideal position to detect and counsel women at risk of disordered mental health in the maternalizatum but requires skills in order to fulfil this role effectively.
- Postnatal mental health and ill-health should be openly discussed with women and their partners in pregnancy, and information made freely available. Rather than frightening people this can allow them realistically to prepare for the many emotional and relationship changes they will experience as they enter parenthood.
- There is a need for further research into all aspects of disordered mental well-being in childbearing women. Medically based studies are likely to have only limited success as mental well-being appears to revolve around emotional, cultural and psychosocial factors.

References

Abramsky, L. 1994: In Abramsky, L. and Chapple, J. (eds), *Prenatal diagnosis: the human side.* London: Chapman and Hall.

Adams, M. 1977: Providing a service. A supplement on parentcraft. *Nursing Mirror* supplement, xii–xiii.

Adams, M., Armstrong-Esther, C., Bryer, R., Duberley, J., Strong, G. and Ward, E. 1981: Trial run. *Nursing Mirror* 153(15), 32–5.

Adams, M. 1989: A study of communications in the labour ward. In *Research and the midwife conference proceedings.* Department of Nursing, University of Manchester.

Allot, S. 1996: PND. Beating the blues. *Telegraph Magazine*, 38.

Allot, H. 1996: Post-traumatic stress disorder may follow childbirth. *British Medical Journal* 313, 28 September.

Anonymous 1993: Postnatal depression. A midwife describes her own experience of a delayed diagnosis. *Midwives Chronicle* 106(1269), 386–7.

Appleby, L., Fox, H., Shaw, M. and Kumar R. 1989: The psychiatrist in the obstetric unit: establishing a liaison service. *British Journal of Psychiatry* 154, 510–15.

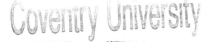

Ball, J. 1989: Postnatal care and adjustment to motherhood. In Robinson, S. and Thomson, A.M. (eds), *Midwives research and childbirth*, Vol. 1. London: Chapman and Hall, 154–74.

Ballard, C., Davis, R. and Dean, C. 1994: Study in postnatal depression in mothers and fathers. In *Recent advances in childbearing and mental health*. Abstracts of the Sixth International Conference of the Marcé Society. *British Journal of Psychiatry* 164, 782–8.

Barnett, B. 1991: *Coping with postnatal depression*. Melbourne, Australia: Lothian Publishing.

Beck, C.T. 1995a: The effect of postpartum depression on maternal–infant interaction: A meta-analysis. *Nursing Research* 44, 289–304.

Beck, C.T. 1995b: Perceptions of nurses' caring by mothers experiencing postpartum depression. *Journal of Obstetric, Gynaecologic and Neonatal Nursing* 24(9), 819–25.

Beck, C. 1996: Postpartum depressed mothers' experiences interacting with their children. *Nursing Research* March–April 45, 2.

Bettes, B. 1988: Maternal depression and motherese: Temporal and intonational features. *Child Development* 59, 1089–96.

Black, T. 1986: *Antenatal education: teaching the teachers*. Report of seminar paper presented at the Health Education Council, London.

Blake, F. 1996: Post-traumatic stress disorder may follow childbirth. *British Medical Journal* 313, 774.

Bohn, D. 1990: Domestic violence in pregnancy: implications for practice. *Journal of Midwifery* 35(2), 86–98.

Brockington, I. and Cox-Roper, A. 1988: The nosology of puerperal mental illness. In Kumar, C. and Brockington, I. (eds), *Motherhood and mental illness*, vol. 2, *Causes and effects*. London: Wright, 13–14.

Bryar, R. 1987: A study of the introduction of the nursing process in a maternity unit. Unpublished Master of Philosophy thesis, Polytechnic of South Bank, London.

Caplan, H., Cogall, S. and Alexander, H. 1989: Maternal depression and the emotional development of the child. *British Journal of Psychiatry* 154, 818–23.

Clarke, M. and Williams, A. 1979: Depression in women after perinatal death. *Lancet* i, 916–17.

Comport, M. 1987: *Towards happy motherhood: understanding postnatal depression*. London: Corgi Books.

Condon, J. 1987: Psychological and physical symptoms during pregnancy; a comparison of male and female expectant parents. *Journal of Reproductive Infant Psychology* 5, 205–13.

Cox, J. 1986: *Postnatal depression: a guide for health professionals*. Edinburgh: Churchill Livingstone.

Cox, A., Sagovsky, R. and Cox, J. 1987: Detection of postnatal depression; development of the ten item Edinburgh postnatal depression scale. *British Journal of Psychiatry* 150, 782–6.

Cox, J. 1988: The life event of childbirth: sociocultural aspects of postnatal depression. In Kumar, C. and Brockington, I. (eds), *Motherhood and mental illness*, vol. 2, *Causes and effects*. London: Wright, 64–75.

Cox, J. 1989: Can postnatal depression be prevented? *Midwife, Health Visitor, and Community Nurse* 25(8), 329.

Cox, J. and Holden, J. (eds) 1994: *Perinatal psychiatry, use and misuse of the Edinburgh Postnatal Depression Scale.* London: Gaskell Royal College of Psychiatrists.

Crockenburg, S. 1986: Are temperamental differences in babies associated in the predictable differences in care giving? In Lerner, J. and Lerner, R. (eds), *Temperament and social interaction during infancy and childhood,* no. 31. San Francisco: Jossey Bass, 53–72.

Dalton, K. 1985: Progesterone prophylaxis used successfully in postnatal depression. *Practitioner* 229, 507–8.

Davis, H. and Fallowfield, L. 1992: *Counselling and communication in health care.* Chichester: John Wiley.

Dennerstein, L., Lehert, P. and Riphagen, F. 1989: Postpartum depression – risk factors. *Journal of Psychosomatic Obstetrics and Gynaecology,* suppl. 10, 53–65.

Department of Health 1976: *Fit for the future.* Court report. London: HMSO.

Department of Health 1978: *First report from the Select Committee on Violence in the Family,* Session 1976/1977 *Violence to children* 28.3.1978. London: HMSO.

Department of Health 1993a: *The health of the nation: key area handbook on mental illness.* London: HMSO.

Department of Health 1993b: *Changing childbirth,* part 1, *the report of the expert group.* London: HMSO.

Dix, C. 1987: *The new mother syndrome: coping with postnatal stress and depression.* London: Unwin.

Dobash, R. and Dobash, R. 1987: Violence towards wives. In Orford, J. (ed.), *Coping with disorder in the family.* London: Croom Helm Beckers.

Dube, R. 1992: Postnatal depression: A community nurse's view. *Bulletin of the Marcé Society* Autumn, 17–20.

Eden, C. 1989: Midwives knowledge and management of postnatal depression. *The Australian Journal of Advanced Nursing* 7, September–November, 35–42.

Elliot, S., Rugg, A., Watson, J. and Brough, D. 1983: Mood changes during pregnancy and after the birth of a child. *British Journal of Clinical Psychology* 22, 295–308.

Elliot, S. 1985: A rationale for psychosocial intervention in the prevention of postnatal depression. Paper presented at the first Women in Psychology conference, Cardiff.

Enkin, M., Marc, J., Keirse, C., Renfrew, M. and Neilson, J. 1995: *A guide to effective care in pregnancy and childbirth.* Oxford: Oxford University Press, 346–7.

Field, T., Healy, B., Goldstein, S. and Guthertz, M. 1990: Behaviour-state matching and synchrony in mother–infant interactions of non depressed versus depressed dyads. *Developmental Psychology* 26, 7–14.

Fisher, J., Stanley, R. and Burrows, G. 1990: Psychological adjustment to caesarean delivery. A review of the evidence. *Journal of Psychosomatic Obstetrics and Gynaecology* 11, 91–106.

Friedman, T. and Gath, D. 1989: The psychiatric consequences of spontaneous abortion. *British Journal of Psychiatry* 155, 810–13.

Goffman, I. 1982: *The presentation of self in everyday life.* London: Pelican Books.

Green, J. 1990a: Is the baby alright and other worries. *Journal of Reproductive Psychology* 8, 225–6.

Green, J. 1990b: Who is unhappy after childbirth? Antenatal and intrapartum correlates from a prospective study. *Journal of Reproductive and Infant Psychology* 8, 175–83.

Green, J., Statham, H. and Snowdon, C. 1994: *Pregnancy: a testing time.* Report of the Cambridge Prenatal Screening study, Centre for Family Research, University of Cambridge, Cambridge.

Gregoire, A., Kumar, R., Everitt, B., Henderson, A. and Studd, J. 1996: Transdermal oestrogen for treatment of severe postnatal depression. *Lancet* 347, April, 930–3.

Hannah, P., Adams, D. and Lee, A. 1992: Links between early postpartum mood and postnatal depression. *British Journal of Psychiatry* 160, 777–80.

Harris, B. 1993: A hormonal component to postnatal depression. *British Journal of Psychiatry* 163, 403–5.

Harvey, I. and McGrath, G. 1988: Psychiatric morbidity in spouses of women admitted to a mother and baby unit. *British Journal of Psychiatry* 152, 506–10.

Henderson, A., Gregoire, A. and Kumar, R. 1991: Treatment of severe postnatal depression with oestriol skin patches. *Lancet* 338: 8167.

Henderson, C. 1984: Influences and interactions surrounding the midwife's decision to rupture the membranes. In *Research and the midwife conference proceedings.* Nursing Research Unit, Kings College, University of London.

Holden, J., Sagovsky, R. and Cox, J. 1989: Counselling in a general practice setting: a controlled study of health visitor intervention in the treatment of postnatal depression. *British Medical Journal* 298, 223–6.

Hutton, E. 1994: What women want from midwives. *British Journal of Midwifery* 2(12), 608.

Jacobson, B., Smith, A. and Whitehead, M. (eds) 1991: *The nation's health: a strategy for the 1990s.* London: King Edward's Fund for London.

Kendall, R. and Zealley, A. 1993: *Companion to psychiatric studies*, vol. 5. Edinburgh: Churchill Livingstone.

Kleiverda, G., Steen, A., Anderson, I., Treffers, P. and Everaerd, W. 1991: Confinement in nulliparous women in the Netherlands: Subjective experiences related to actual events and to postpartum well-being. *Journal of Reproductive and Infant Psychology* 9, 195–213.

Kumar, C. and Brockington, I. 1988: *Motherhood and mental illness*, vol. 2, *causes and effects.* London: Wright.

Kumar, R. 1990: An overview of postpartum psychiatric disorders. *NAACOGS Clinical Issues in Perinatal and Women's Health Nursing* I(3), 351–8.

Kumar, R., Marks, M. and Jackson, K. 1995: Prevention and treatment of postnatal psychiatric disorders. *British Journal of Midwifery* 3(6), 314–17.

Lambert, T.W. and Lambert, W. 1964: The social significance of attitudes. In *Social Psychology*, vol. 4. Foundations of modern psychology series. London: Prentice Hall, 50–1.

Laryea, M. 1989: Midwives and mothers' perceptions of motherhood. In Robinson, S. and Thomson, A. (eds), *Midwives research and childbirth*, vol. 1. London: Chapman and Hall, 176–89.

Macleod Clark, J. 1981: Communication in nursing. *Nursing Times* 77(1), 12–18.

Marks, M., Wieck, A., Checkley, S. and Kumar, R. 1991: Life stress and postpartum psychosis. A preliminary report. *British Journal of Psychiatry* 158(10), 45–9.

Marteau, T., Slack, J., Kidd, J. and Shaw, R. 1992a: Presenting a routine screening test in antenatal care: practice observed. *Public Health* 106, 131–41.

Marteau, T., Johnson, M. and Kidd, J. 1992b: Psychological models in predicting uptake of prenatal screening. *Psychology and Health* 6, 13–22.

McClary, M. and Stokoe, B. 1995: A multidisciplinary approach to postnatal depression. *Health Visitor* 68(4), 141–3.

McIntosh, J. 1993: Postpartum depression: women's self-seeking behaviour and perceptions of cause. *Journal of Advanced Nursing* 18(2), 178–84.

McKay, S. 1991: Shared power: The essence of humanized childbirth. *Pre- and Peri-Natal Psychology* 5(4), 283–95.

Menage, J. 1996: Post-traumatic stress disorder may follow childbirth. *British Medical Journal* 313, 28 September.

Methven, R. 1989: Recording an obstetric history or relating to a pregnant woman? A study of the antenatal booking interview. In Robinson, S. and Thomson, A. (eds), *Midwives research and childbirth*, vol. 1. London: Chapman and Hall, 42–70.

Meyer, J. and Wallace, V. 1995: Mothers' help Nursing Times 3M National nursing awards. *Nursing Times* 91(50), 42–3.

Milgrom, J. 1994: Mother–infant interaction in postpartum depression, and early intervention programme. *The Australian Journal of Advanced Nursing* 11(4), 29–37.

Mills, M., Puckering, C., Pound, A. and Cox, A. 1985: What is it about depressed mothers that influences their children's functioning? In Stevenson, J. (ed.), *Recent research in developmental psychopathology.* Oxford: Pergamon Press, 11–17.

Murray, L. 1988: Effects of postnatal depression on infant development: direct studies of early mother–infant interactions. In Kumar, R. and Brockington, I. (eds), *Motherhood and mental illness*, vol. 2, *causes and effects.* London: Wright, 161.

Murray, L., Cooper, P.J. and Stein, A. 1991: Postnatal depression and infant development. *British Medical Journal* 309, 378–9.

Murray, D., Cox, D., Chapman, G. and Jones, P. 1995: Childbirth: life event or start of long term difficulty? Further data from the Stoke on Trent controlled study of post natal depression. *British Journal of Psychiatry* 166(5), 595–600.

Murray, L., Stanley, C., Hooper, R., King, F. and Fiori-Cowley, A. 1996: The role of infant factors in postnatal depression and mother–infant interactions. *Developmental Medicine and Child Neurology* 38, 109–19.

Nicholson, P. 1990: Understanding postnatal depression: A mother centred approach. *Journal of Advanced Nursing* 15, 689–95.

Niven, C. 1992: *Psychological care for families: before, during and after birth.* Oxford: Butterworth-Heinemann, 241.

O'Hara, M. and Zekoski, E. 1988: Postpartum depression: a comprehensive review. In Kumar, C. and Brockington, I. (eds), *Motherhood and mental illness*, vol. 2, *causes and effects.* London: Wright, 17–57.

Okpala, D. 1991: Preventing postnatal depression. *Nursing Standard* 5(36), 32–4.

Page, L. 1993: Education for practice. *MIDIRS Midwifery Digest* 3, 256.

Paradice, K. 1995: Postnatal depression: a normal response to motherhood? *British Journal of Midwifery* 3(12), 632–5.

Pease, K. 1974: *Communication with and without words.* Vernon Scott Associates.

Pitts, F. 1995: Comrades in adversity: the group approach. *Health Visitor* 68(4), 144–5.

Prince, J. and Adams, M. 1977: *Minds, mothers and midwives. The psychology of childbirth*. Edinburgh: Churchill Livingstone.

Prince, J. and Adams, M. 1987: *The psychology of childbirth – an introduction for mothers and midwives*. Edinburgh: Churchill Livingstone.

Raphael-Leff, J. 1991: *Psychological processes of childbearing*. London: Chapman and Hall.

Resnick, P.J. 1969: Child murder by parents. A psychiatric view of filicide. *American Journal of Psychiatry* 126, 325–34.

Resnick, P.J. 1970: Murder of the new-born: a psychiatric review of neonaticide. *American Journal of Psychiatry* 126, 1414–20.

Riley, D. 1995: *Perinatal mental health, a source book for professionals*. Oxford: Radcliffe Medical Press.

Roberts, D. 1984: Non-verbal communication. Popular and unpopular patients. In Faulkner, A. (ed.), *Communication*. Edinburgh: Churchill Livingstone, 12–17.

Schaper, A., Rooney, B., Kay, N. and Silva, P. 1994: Use of the Edinburgh postnatal depression scale to identify postpartum depression in a clinical setting. *Journal of Reproductive Medicine* 139(8), 620–4.

Seeley, S., Murray, L. and Cooper, P. 1996: The outcome for mothers and babies of health visitor intervention. *Health Visitor* 69(4), 135–8.

Sharp, D. 1989: Emotional disorders during pregnancy and the puerperium – a longitudinal prospective study in primary care. *Marcé Society Bulletin* Spring.

Sherr, L. 1995: *Psychology of pregnancy and childbirth*. Oxford: Blackwell Science.

Stein, A., Gath, D., Bucher, J., Bond, A., Day, A. and Cooper, P. 1991: The relationship between postnatal depression and mother–child interaction. *British Journal of Psychiatry* 158, 46–52.

Stern, G. and Kruckona, L. 1983: Multidisciplinary perspectives on postpartum depression: an anthropological critique. *Social Science and Medicine* 17, 1027–41.

Thorpe, K., Dragonas, T. and Golding, J. 1992: The effects of psychosocial factors on the emotional well-being of women during pregnancy: A cross cultural study of Britain and Greece. *Journal of Reproductive and Infant Psychology* 10, 191–204.

Thurtle, V. 1995: Postnatal depression. The relevance of sociological approaches. *Journal of Advanced Nursing* 22, 416–24.

Tylden, E. 1990: Post traumatic stress disorder in obstetrics. Paper presented at the Fifth International Conference of Childbearing and Mental Health. Marcé Society, University of York, UK.

Ussher, J. 1992: Reproductive rhetoric and the blaming of the body. In Nicholson, P. and Ussher, J. (eds), *The psychology of woman's health and health care*. Basingstoke: Macmillan Press.

Van der Meer, Y., Loendersloot, E. and Van Loenen, A. 1984: The effect of high dose progesterone in postpartum depression. *Journal of Psychosomatic Obstetrics and Gynaecology* 3, 67–8.

Watson, J., Elliot, S., Rugg, A. and Brough, D. 1984: Psychiatric disorder in pregnancy and the first postnatal year. *British Journal of Psychiatry* 144, 454–62.

Williams, A., Ware, J. and Donald, C. 1981: A model of mental health, life events and social supports applicable to General Populations. *Journal of Health and Social Behaviour* 22, December, 324–36.

Wilson, P. 1990: *Antenatal teaching. A guide to theory and practice.* London: Faber and Faber.

Wheatley, S. 1996: Antenatal sources of social support as predictors of early postnatal depression, positive affect, and negative affect. Partners in parenthood – Who needs them? Unpublished paper, University of Leicester.

Further reading

Dix, C. 1987: *The new mother syndrome: coping with postnatal stress and depression.* London: Unwin Paperbacks.

Kumar, R. 1990: An overview of postpartum psychiatric disorders. *NAACOGS Clinical Issues in Perinatal and Women's Health Nursing* 1(3), 351–8.

Kumar, R., Marks, M. and Jackson, K. 1995: Prevention and treatment of postnatal psychiatric disorders. *British Journal of Midwifery* 3(6), 314–17.

Meyer, J. and Wallace, V. 1995: Mothers' help Nursing Times 3M. National nursing awards. *Nursing Times* 91(50), 42–3.

Niven, C. 1992: *Psychological care for families: before, during and after birth.* Oxford: Butterworth-Heinemann.

Raphael-Leff, J. 1991: *Psychological processes of childbearing.* London: Chapman and Hall.

Riley, D. 1995: *Perinatal mental health, a source book for professionals.* Oxford: Radcliffe Medical Press.

Index